All of Their Kind

By Peter Gurney

To all those wonderful vets who love them as we do,
value them as we do and care for them as we do.

First Published in 2002 by

Peter Gurney

In collaboration with

The Winking Cavy Store
PO Box 68
Whitley Bay
Tyne & Wear
NE25 9YW

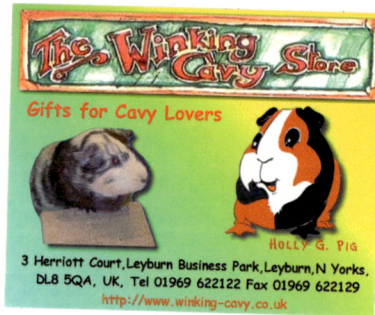

The Winking Cavy Store
Gifts for Cavy Lovers
HOLLY G. PIG
3 Herriott Court, Leyburn Business Park, Leyburn, N Yorks,
DL8 5QA, UK, Tel 01969 622122 Fax 01969 622129
http://www.winking-cavy.co.uk

ISBN ……..

Editor: John Ogbourne

Cartoons: Phil Anderton

Photography: Peter Gurney

Peter Gurney's website:
http://www.cavy.fslife.co.uk/home.html

ISBN 0-9542505-0-8

9 780954 250508

Foreword.

This is the book I have always wanted to write for it tells the tale, not only of how these adorable creatures took over my life but introduced me to some absolutely wonderful human beings and I want to tell their story as well. However, one of the reasons these animals have become so much part of my life is because I believe and still believe, that the veterinary profession fails them, dismally. To leave this part of my story untold would be a failure on my part to tell the whole truth.

In the main the problem is not with individual vets but with the system by which their profession is regulated and the lack lustre of politicians to take the concerns of small animals owners seriously.

My admiration for skills of the many open minded vets with whom I have worked is boundless. I'm pleased to say that more of them are turning to the Cambridge Cavy Trust and myself when they happen to be stymied by a piggy problem. That is all we ask for, for if we are good then it is because we asked those who had the knowledge that we lacked!

Peter Gurney

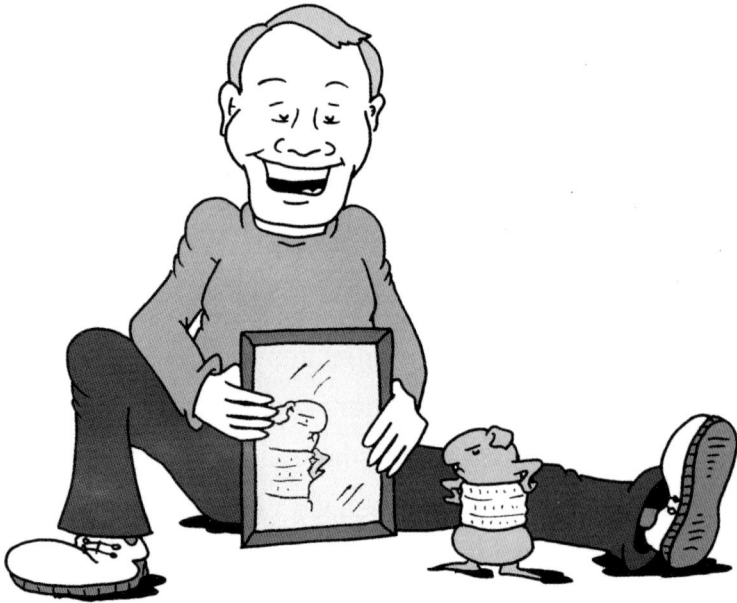

Chapter one.

Criminal activities.

Her cries awoke me, high pitched and piercing. The red glowing digits of my bedside clock told me that it was two fifty three in the morning. The effects of the anaesthetic spray had obviously worn off, and she must have been scratching at those raw open lesions.

I roused myself, and swung my legs over the edge of my bed and sat there a few seconds, waiting for my sleep fuddled brain to send the necessary messages to the rest of my body to make it stand up. When the connections were made, I hobbled across to my writing desk and fumbled for my glasses, cursing myself for the umpteenth time for not hanging them up on the purpose made hook that I had carefully fixed to the bed post closest to my pillow over a year earlier.

I am not at my tactile best in the wee small hours just after my slumbers have been disturbed so the noise caused by my fumbling fingers in the clutter of the writing paraphernalia set off a few of the eighty guinea pigs that I share my home with. They obviously thought that perhaps the 'piggy person' was going to give them an early breakfast. There was sufficient light from my electric fly catcher, high up on one wall for me to manage, so I had no intention of switching on the main light for that would have set the lot off!

I 'shushed' them in the loudest whisper I could hiss, which was a mistake for a few more joined in the chorus.

"Oh, shut up, you lot," I said, out loud, giving up the struggle to keep a low profile. "Go back to sleep," I called over my shoulder, as I headed out for the kitchen, picking up my dressing gown on the way and throwing it on. It wasn't a cold night but I figured that the retched patient in my kitchen had suffered quite enough already without being confronted with the sight of a strange, naked sixty one year old man looming over her!

She went by the odd name of 'Tiswas', I had been told, and she and her two eight-day-old babies had been brought to me earlier that evening.

I looked down into the large plastic Curver box in the corner of my kitchen by the immersion heater. Not for the first time since these wonderful little creatures had come into my life, I was torn between conflicting emotions of anger, the most intense love and respect, frustration, and deep gratitude.

There she was, crouched in the typical hunch backed, suckling position that all lactating sows take when they feed their young, her two babies firmly attached to each one of her nipples, enjoying the their mother's warm milk.

I stood and watched in wonderment, for every so often Tiswas twitched and winced as spasms shot through the muscles of her back in reaction to the pain caused by those terrible open lesions. However, she held her position, her priority, the giving of nourishment to her babies and not the suffering she was enduring.

My anger was at the veterinary surgeon that was the direct cause of this pain. My love and respect was inspired by this animal's total devotion to her young. My frustration was at my not being able to ease her suffering quickly enough to my satisfaction, and my gratitude was to all of her kind for bringing so much joy into my life.

There was a bonus that sometimes I am inclined to forget. These adorable creatures have also brought some absolutely wonderful people into my life, who have been a very healthy antidote to a strong streak of misanthrope which has served me very well in dealing with my own species during the past sixty three years in this world.

However, loving these people as much as I do has not blunted the edge of my wariness of my fellow human beings. If anything, it has honed it up very nicely. Now, when I take on the politicians, the many lettered and those that look the other way in the face of human indifference, deviousness and down right evil intent, I feel that I am fighting for my human friends as well as my animal ones.

"And who pulled your chains, may I ask?" this was to my then, current free ranger guinea pigs, Dusty and Dennis, whom, always with an eye for the main chance, had wondered to the front of their open fronted pen under the fridge and oven. They peered up at me, blinking in the bright light, wearing their 'what have you got for us?' faces. It usually worked but I figured that this little lady's needs were greater than theirs.

"In you go, you bums," I said, shushing them back inside their quarters and placing a couple of bricks across the front that I always keep handy for the purpose. The last thing I wanted was a pair of very inquisitive boars under my feet at a time like this.

I waited till the babies were sated then very gently lifted Tiswas out of the box and placed her on a towel on my kitchen table.

She was certainly a mess, bald, apart from some hair around her jaws and on the top of her head, and a small amount on her rump. Though sow guinea pigs, like many mammals, can lose hair through hormonal deficiencies when they are pregnant, this little lady was suffering from a serious fungal skin condition, which was causing the hair loss and intense irritation and pain.

When she had arrived, I had immediately sprayed her with Xylocane, an over the counter anaesthetic, formulated for use on human beings suffering from dental pain or the pain from minor wounds. Though this was only a palliative and was in no way anti fungal, it would numb the lesions and stop her from making them worse by scratching at them.

It hadn't taken long for the Xylocane to take effect, after which I smothered her in aloe Vera gel. This is not only mildly anti fungal, it is very soothing to the skin and I was hoping that this, in combination with the anaesthetic, would see her through the night. I had obviously been wrong.

"Sorry little lass but it's the waistcoat treatment for you," I told, as she crouched there, fearful and suspicious.

I knew that I would have to do it in the morning when I had been working on her the previous evening so it just meant bringing it forward a few hours. The waistcoat treatment is simply a way of covering up the lesions by making a waistcoat out of Tubigrip bandage. This is a tubular, elasticized, surgical support bandage that is normally used upon strain injuries in the ankles, knees, thighs or elbows of human beings. I always use the knee size, which is tight enough to prevent the patient from wriggling it off, but not so tight as to restrict the respiration.

Depending upon the size of the guinea pig, a length between seven and ten inches is cut off and a couple of small holes are cut out, an inch to an inch and a half from one end for the front legs to go through.

It only took me a couple of minutes to make up the waistcoat, splay it wide on my fingers, slip it over her head then roll it back down over her body. This effectively covered the open lesions. I quickly put her back into the Curver box and stood by, tense for I knew exactly what was about to happen. As soon as I let go of her she jumped and bucked like a wild stallion trying to unseat a rider in a wild west show. They always did. It's very traumatic for a guinea pig to suddenly find itself wearing a garment of any kind when it came into this world with a perfectly adequate coat of it's own!

The babies, wisely, kept a low profile, huddling in a far corner of the box while mother was acting so peculiarly. I put some cucumber pieces, grass and parsley into the box, which at first she would grab between jumps then gradually she calmed down and began to eat with a will, twitching now and again. It usually takes about five minutes or so for a guinea pig to accept the situation and from there on out it will totally ignore the waistcoat.

"It's all for your own good," I reassured her as she was at the height of her leaping.

How many times have I said that to a guinea pig to whom I had had to do something unpleasant but that was a necessary part of it's treatment? I remember thinking about my mother that morning, who had died at the grand old age of ninety about eight months earlier. If she was somewhere up there, looking down on me, she certainly would have known where those words had come from for she had said them to me so many times when she had been patching me up after yet one more fall when I was a small boy. If I remember rightly, she also regularly accused me of being deformed, in that I possessed two left feet, and was incapable of looking where I was going!

I made myself a cup of tea, pulled back the bricks from the front of the lad's quarters and invited them out. Dusty was the first, and immediately sat up and begged for a portion of the cucumber that he knew was in the offing. This pair could scent cucumber if you cut into one a mile off! As I leaned down to give him his portion, Dennis hastened out for his share. The pair of them immediately rushed back into their quarters where they settled down in opposite corners, eyeing each other, guardedly, as they gobbled down their treats. These two brothers were the very best of friends and I had never seen the slightest sign of any aggression between them. However, when it came to cucumber, then that was serious business. The number one rule was that your bit was yours and that his was his, end of debate!

I reflected that since Tiswas had come to me seven hours earlier, I had committed two criminal offences, punishable by a very heavy fine. I had treated an animal that was not my own, so had broken the 1966 veterinary surgeon's act, which makes it a criminal offence for anyone, not a qualified veterinary surgeon to treat animals other than their own. I had also broken the 1994 veterinary medicines act in that I had used medicines on an animal, not my own, that was not licensed for use upon animals.

The veterinary surgeon who had the exclusive legal right to treat her, had misdiagnosed her condition and prescribed drugs that were not only totally ineffective against the fungal skin condition that she was suffering from, but that were also a danger to her lactating babies.

This fact, of course, is of no concern of the law. We have all been told that many times. The law is their to protect animals against people like myself and others, far more skilled than I am, who have not had the 'benefit' of five years training in one of our wonderful veterinary colleges!

The only problem is, of course, that there is no counter balancing law that protects animals from incompetent veterinary surgeons. There are statutory procedures to make complaints against incompetent veterinary surgeons but as they are policed by the very people that are the cause of the complaints, the veterinary authorities, they are, like all self regulatory rules, a sick joke! Even if they did come out and support a complaint against a vet, by the time they had come to the end of their lengthy deliberations, the animal would be long dead. As for any kind of effective sanction being taken against the vet concerned, long experience as taught me, and many who have jumped through these official hoops, that blue moons are very rare!

The sky had that pre dawn tinge to it when I finally sloped back off to bed that morning. It didn't take me long to slip off to sleep, Call it contentment, with a touch of resolution, which gave me peace of mind. I left Tiswas resting easy in her waistcoat, her babies snuggled up to her, and I was more confident that I was going to undo the damage done to her by the professional. The laws of the land, and those with such blind faith in professional advice that had framed them, had declared that I should leave the business to a vet because he had letters after his name and I did not, were, in reality the cause of this retched animal's suffering.

Once more I had intervened and managed to ease the suffering of an animal and maybe saved the lives of her young. This was happening more frequently, and as time passed and my expertise increased, my resolution to beat the powerful odds stacked against me simply grew stronger.

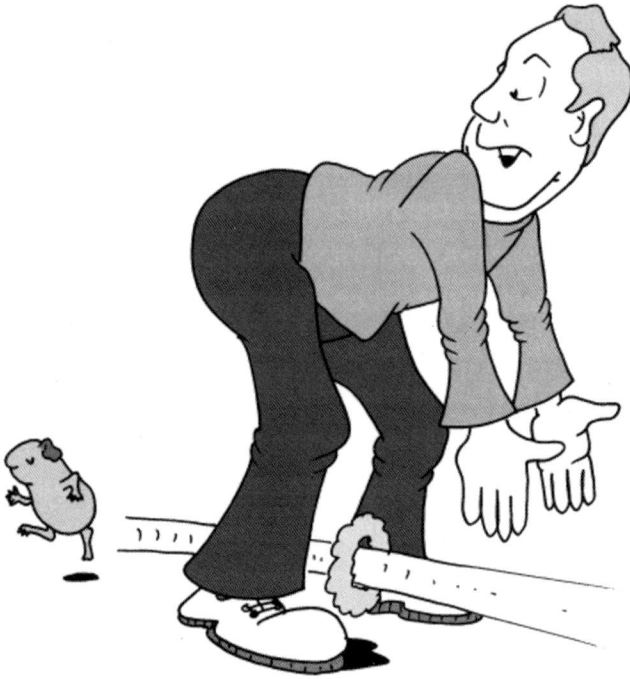

Chapter two.

Genesis.

It had all begun fifteen years earlier with a small black guinea pig called Bubble. I had just moved into a new flat where I still live in Clapham, South London and had just come to the end of yet another disastrous love affair. To ice my cake, I had been made redundant after thirteen years of steady employment!

The flat was fine but I could have done without the other two problems! I can't pretend that the love affair fiasco was a surprise for as a twice married and divorced man who had been in and out of love more times than he cared to think about, such things had become kind of routine! I would feel deflated for a while, wondering where I had gone wrong that time, swear to give up women for good, then the old Adam would get the upper hand in me and off I would go on the familiar merry go round again. By that time I guess it was a case of there being no fool like an old fool!

The loss of the job really did come as a body blow for I enjoyed it and the company was a good one to work for. It was a couple of months after I had been made redundant that I got the flat and by that time I had managed to get another job, driving a truck for a scaffolding company.

I still don't know how I managed to reach the age of forty eight, from the age of eighteen, which was the last time an animal was in my life, bereft of beasties! I always adored them and was brought up in a home that was never without an animal of some kind or another. Both my parents taught we children to respect and care for animals but in my case I am certain that that it was as much a matter of nature as nurture.

I still cannot see a dog walking along a street without saying hello to it and not wanting to be friends, be it noble pedigree or the most mixed up mongrel upon four legs. Very early on in life I found that the company of animals to be far more enjoyable than that of my own kind.

However, the fact remains, that until the first guinea pig came into my life, for thirty years I had managed to cope without an animal. Was it because I felt that I had grown out of them, that they were things of my childhood? Possibly, and if it was then it only goes to show that I was a young fool long before I became an old one!

I do know why I chose a guinea pig. I presumed it would be happy by itself in a cage while I was out at work all day, unlike a dog, which just shows how ignorant I was of the species at that time. I didn't even think of a cat for I am simply not a cat person, though I do think that they are very elegant, noble creatures.

I picked up my first guinea pig from a pet shop in Shepherds Bush, not far from where I was working at the time. She was a small black sow who was housed in a pen, surrounded by a bunch of very lively rabbits. I was immediately attracted by her sleek smooth shiny coat but I think that I also felt a little sorry for her, out numbered by animals that were not of her species and that were far more boisterous than she was.

As, when I was a child, I had been subjected to bullying I felt empathy with Bubble. The name had been at the back of my mind before I even set eyes on her. I was told that she was three months old but in the light of fifteen years experience of both guinea pigs and pet shops that sell them, I am now sure that she must have been closer to six months.

I had brought a cage and felt very mother hennish about my new acquisition as I prepared it for it's new tenant when I got home that night. After much scrabbling about in the box that the pet shop had put Bubble in, I managed to capture her and put her into the cage, which I then placed under the hand basin in my bathroom. Why I abandoned her to the bathroom had something to do with the mind-set that guinea pigs shouldn't be indoors, which prevailed at that time. They lived outdoors in hutches, usually at the bottom of the garden. Well, that's the way it was done and the way that books told you that it should be done. Little did I know that I was going to have to write a few books of my own, in the not too distant future, to dispel that stupid notion. This wee animal was to be, of course, the quintessential cause of my subsequent 'criminal' career!

Lots of things that I was brought up to believe were right because they had always been done that way, I no longer believe are, as a direct result of living with guinea pigs. Lots of people and institutions that I was brought up to respect, I no longer respect, as a direct result of living with guinea pigs. It may have taken me a long time to cotton on to the many rotten ways that the establishment operates, and how to fight it by playing it at it's own game, but I have the humble guinea pig to thank for my eventual enlightenment. So let's hear it, three cheers for the wee beasties!

I resisted the temptation to keep checking up on Bubble, leaving her alone to her own devices so that she could settle in for herself. When I went in first thing in the morning and saw her peering out of through the bars of her cage, I had my first lesson in the wrong way to do it. I just felt that the cage was far too small, and the mere fact that it was a cage was all wrong.

The space under the sink was a little larger than the cage so I blocked it off, lined the floor with paper and wood shavings, and fitted it with a water bottle and feed bowl and put bubble into it. I threw in some fresh grass and went off to work.

When I came home that evening I had my second lesson in guinea pig handling and husbandry. It was that as escape artists, guinea pigs could teach Houdini a trick or two! The piece of wooden shelving that I had wedged in place, and reinforced by placing a heavy toolbox in front of it to block Bubble in had been pushed open at one end. The gap that this had made was so small that I was amazed that she could have got through it but she had for she was nowhere inside her enclosure. However, she hadn't gone far and I quickly found her, crouched behind the toilet pedestal, and this is when the fun started!

Ignorant, as I was in the ways of these agile wily beasties, she avoided my grasping hands with ease and graceful finesse. The piggy person was about to be taught another lesson!

She was off and out of the open bathroom doorway and down the hallway to the living room before I could even stand up and turn round. I didn't panic, and decided to go in for a wee bit of lateral thinking by calmly following her into the living room, closing the door to the hallway behind me, then walking across and pulling the kitchen door too.

"Right, young lady, silly games time is it, eh!" I said confident that having confined her to this one room, the battle between man and beast would swiftly result in a victory for the man in question and defeat for the beast! After all it was my territory, I was reasonably fit and agile, and much bigger than it was. It's funny the way that the 'mighty' set themselves up for their own falls with such confidence!

She immediately begun by giving me a thorough grounding in guinea pig evasive techniques, which I am sure would be worthy of study by any crack army unit. Every time I cornered her or thought that I had trapped her under a chair, the bunk bed that I had at that time, beneath the T.V. stand or in the corner by the small chest of draws, she shot left, right, and a couple of times, just to rub my nose in my own inadequacy, between my legs!

I eventually did manage to capture her but she made me pay the price for it with a grazed arm and a considerable lowering of any expectancy that I may have had of becoming a successful hunter of animals, wild or domestic! What any 'fly on the wall' observer would have made of the sight of a heavily booted, middle aged man, clad in his dirty working clothes, blundering about in hot pursuit of a graceful, sleek animal, is patently clear; guinea pig ten, human being, zilch! They would certainly have learned a few new words, not in the English dictionary for during the chase I was delving deep into my vast reservoir of naval language that I keep by me whenever I am making a complete ass of myself!

However, any anger I may have felt at having been so humiliated fell away when I finally held Bubble up in my hands and looked into her little face. She looked as any animal that had been hounded in that way would look, terrified. I could feel her rapidly increased respiration and she looked resigned to her fate.

My heart went out to her, and I nestled her into the nape of my neck, murmuring quietly, in the way that I had often heard mothers with small babies when they were trying to comfort them after picking them up from a fall. This child of mine struggled briefly then gradually calmed down.

"You and I have got to sort things out between us," I said, at length, as I held her nose to nose. "I'm the boss in this neck of the woods. This is my home, I pay the rent, pay for your food and will soon be making you a proper home of your own."

As a statement of the facts they were fine but as a reflection of the utter poverty of mind of the man laying them down, they were very illuminating! The animal was not there by it's own choice but by mine and for my pleasure. In short, I owed it; it didn't owe me!

I reinforced the length of shelving in front of her bathroom quarters with a couple of bricks and popped her back in.

"What are we going to do with you, Miss Bubble?" I asked, as I lay on my back in the bath about an hour later, with a tummy full after my evening meal but a very empty mind. Well, it was empty is so far as solving the problem of how I was going to provide for Bubble what I considered to be adequate housing. The only conclusion that I had reached was that I wanted her in my living room. I wish I cold say that there was a eureka moment in my bath, I did have one, but that occurred as I was driving my truck through the madness of the morning rush hour a few days later.

I had, by this time, brought a book about the care of guinea pigs. Like most of them at that time, it was full of total nonsense, and it included that cardinal sin of stating that you could safely house a rabbit and a guinea pig together. However, there was at least one bit of good advice, and that was that it was best to leave your guinea pig to it's own devices for a few days, giving it a chance to get used to it's new surrounding in it's own time. This made a lot of sense to me so I did just that, while I pondered on the whys and wherefores of the kind of quarters that I needed and where I would site them in my living room.

It was a single 'bumble,' which is the term used for one of the neat, dry oblong pellets that guinea pigs excrete that was eventually to lead to my eureka moment. This delightful term, to describe guinea pig number ones is not of my own coining but of the wife of Michael Bond, who wrote the charming Olga de Polga books. Guinea pigs are very prolific in the production of these pellets, and they do tend to get into pockets or get secreted about the clothing of those who own these animals.

I was stuck in the usual traffic jam into town, and reaching down into the pocket of my duffle jacket for some change, out came a bumble with the coins. I smiled, and thought fondly of my little flat mate in my bathroom back home. I remembered that it had been a very cold night when I was cleaning out the piggy quarters the night before so I had put on my duffle jacket when I had took the debris from the cleaning down into the bins downstairs. Somehow a bumble had found it's way into the pocket.

Thoughts had been tumbling about my brain of cages, pens, and even at one time a wooden hutch, then suddenly, shortly after discovering the bumble, the eureka moment came. It had reminded me of the fact that even when it came to cleaning out Bubble's quarters, there was no odour from either bumbles or urine. I gave Bubble a get out clause as soon as the new idea came into my head!

'Even if she couldn't be house trained,' I thought, 'Why couldn't she just live free range?' no matter how prolific she was pellet-wise, what's a few bumbles between friends! The only fear I had was that perhaps I would tread on her if both she and I didn't watch where we were going.

By the end of the day I had it very clear in my mind's eye. There would have to be quarters made for her with her water bottle, bowl and bedding but they could be open fronted so that she could come and go as she pleased.

I decided to leave the work until the following week-end for I would have to make sure that any electric wires were covered up for I had already learned that the guinea pig nibble test had to be tried on every conceivable object that Bubble came across. She was already producing some very artistic filigree work on the skirting board that ran along the back of her quarters in the bathroom. If she decided to try the same thing on live electric wires, 250 volts at the rate of 15 amps would be a very unpleasant way for her to exit this world!

On the Friday evening before the quarters were made, Bubble, who had not budged, voluntarily from her bathroom quarters since the day she had arrived, decided to do a bit of exploring and find out where the piggy person lived.

I was sitting in my easy chair, my head in a book. This meant that my back was towards the hallway and the first that I was aware of her presence was a black flash to my right, as bubble made a dash for small table that stood against the kitchen wall.

When guinea pigs explore new territory in the shape of a new room, they keep close to the walls and if they do have to cross an open space, then they do it in top gear.

I immediately did my statue impression, fearful that the slightest movement from me would send Bubble scurrying back into the bathroom. She sat there, watchful, paws hovering over the panic button, for what seemed like an age. Then, first she sniffed, then she licked, and finally she did some serious nibble testing of the skirting board.

I smiled and relaxed a wee bit. Then, almost as though she was taking her cue from me, she too seemed to relax for she began to thoroughly groom herself. By the liberal use of her tongue, fore and back paws, every nook and cranny of her body was worked upon. I think it was as she was combing her snout in a kind of frantic face washing action, that another tie was made to her species that would bind me to them for as long as I took breath. Up until that moment, I think that there had always been a nagging doubt that perhaps it was the novelty of it all that was captivating me but I was now certain that this was a life long love affair. My American friends would call the cleaning behavior of guinea pigs cute but that wasn't sufficient to describe the great fountain of warmth that I felt at the sight of a guinea pig grooming for the first time in my life. It is so domestic, so thorough and hey, it is something that the human animal has to do as well!

When it comes to the history of the ladies in my life I have always thought that the words that the dying Othello says as the end of the play are particularly relevant. 'Write me down as one who loved well but not too wisely."

Now, what I felt was something far deeper than anything I had ever felt before. I am certain that a part of it was a deep paternalism that had, up until that time, lain dormant. I had fallen in love again but perhaps this time, wisely. The past fourteen years of my life have proved that this foolish man has gained some wisdom in love at long last!

I was deeply honoured that Bubble had finally plucked up courage to enter the piggy person's domain. Even though she suddenly took to her heels and flew back down the hallway at some slight movement I must have made, I felt that we had made a giant step forward in our relationship. Also, my fanciful imagination went into overdrive, telling me that this was Bubble's way of checking the place out before she moved in!

I made my first of many trips down to the local DIY store, the ex jazz drummer, the right on, cool cat! Never the less, there I was, clutching my little piece of paper with my carefully made measurements written on it, my flexible rule, and even a pencil behind my ear just like my dad used to have! That it should come to this! What was even sadder was the fact that I thoroughly enjoyed the experience and found the place a veritable treasure-trove of goodies!

Returning home with the necessary pieces of wooden battening, and a length of chipboard to make the base and sides of the enclosure, I felt very satisfied with myself and there was that novel feeling in my soul, a nesting instinct!

It took about two hours, judicial use of the Elastoplast tin, and the expenditure of a fair amount of my naval vocabulary before the work was completed to my satisfaction. The main problem was that the tolerances allowed in my measurements were all out, which was more likely due to my lousy mathematics than my eyesight or the tools that I used!

Job completed, I sat back on my haunches and admired my handiwork.

"Hm, what do you think of that, dad?" I asked my long dead father. "Not bad for a bodger.eh!"

My father, a skilled carpenter by trade, gave up very early on in our relationship, any hopes that I would follow in his footsteps.

"Not bad. Not bad at all," I relied for him then I got to my feet and went out into the bathroom to see what the most important critic of my handiwork would think of it!

When I put Bubble in her new quarters she immediately buried herself under the hay and adamantly refused to come out.

"Well, I think it's a pretty good home," I said, settling down to watch from the comfort of my armchair, all high dudgeon and 'so there!'

For a few minutes the pair of us retained our sulks. It was Bubble who broke the impasse, her natural curiosity over coming her indignity at having been moved from her bathroom quarters. The hay began to tremble, lifted, then a little black snout poked out from beneath.

It was statue time again for me, of course, for I wanted her to be absolutely confident that I was not going to lay hands on her once more.

Her head turned this way and that, and there was a great deal of sniffing going on. Gradually, she crawled out, and I begun busting a gut, trying to gag the giggle that was gurgling to the surface. Around her shoulders was a very fetching wreath of hay and I mused that a matching grass skirt was all that she need to complete the Hawaiian ensemble!

The tour of inspection that followed, reminded me of my navy days when the first lieutenant did his Saturday morning rounds, wearing white gloves to touch here and there to detect the slightest sign of dirt or dust. It was thorough, and at several junctures, very critical. She obviously didn't think a lot of the way the shavings were arranged at the front of the quarters for she spent a considerable length of time kicking them out onto the carpet. The food and water bottle were fine but she didn't like the smooth beveled edge of the hard wood beading that abutted the wall at the back of her quarters. Apparently, it needed a lot of guinea pig carving to bring it up to the rigorous standards that Bubble used to!

My problem was that I had been thinking like a human being. I thought a smooth surface would be more pleasing and less dangerous to my flat mate. She simply took one look at it and no doubt thought to herself, "Oh my God, I'm living with a Philistine." She gave the beading some preliminary nibbles to get the measure of the texture of the material that she had to work upon, and then decided that she would get back to it later. Oh, and how she did for after a few days the smooth wood had been carved into a design, which was I can only describe as a splintered hemp rope. I thought it was a mess but what can you expect from a Philistine with no artistic taste what so ever!

Not to my surprise, on that first night she didn't leave her quarters at all, after I had gone to sleep. If she did, then she was very careful not to leave any droppings as evidence of her nocturnal wondering.

When I woke up the following morning, I opened my eyes and looked across towards Bubble's new quarters, I could see her lying on her side, half mooned, a familiar position for some guinea pigs to sleep in. I couldn't see if her eyes were open for she had her back to me, not that this would have told me if she was awake or not for guinea pigs can and do sleep with their eyes open or closed.

I usually get up as soon as I wake up in the morning but that morning I just stayed put, watching the rise and fall of Bubble's sides as she breathed, easily. I felt a great surge of contentment within myself that this wee animal was confident enough to feel at ease with the huge, noisy, clumsy creature that had come into her life.

She was the first of so many that I was too lose my heart to, Little did I know that in a few week's time she would be dead, killed by the ignorance of an incompetent veterinary surgeon!

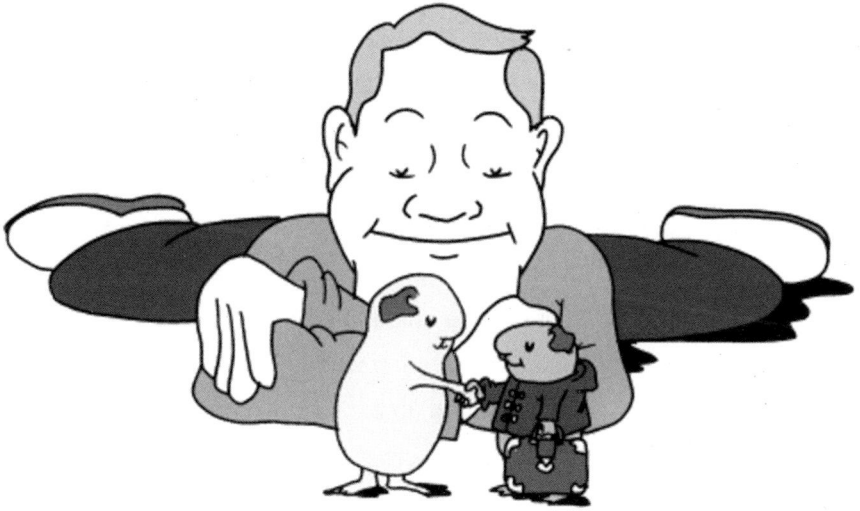

Chapter three.

A death in the family.

Bubble had come to me in late February and one month later Squeak arrived. Though Bubble seemed happy enough and was now not the nervous little creature that she had been when she had arrived, I just felt that she needed company. Guinea pigs are pack animals in the wild and though they have been domesticated in this country for over three hundred years, in evolutionary terms this was nothing. Even the dog, which has lived with man since he was living in caves is still a pack animal.

I had read that guinea pigs were eaten by the natives of South America but as I too was a carnivore at this time, I was not too deeply shocked. However, within a year of living with guinea pigs I changed a lifetime's habit and became a vegetarian. I now have to hold my nose when I pass a butcher's shop for the smell of dead meat of any kind turns my stomach. I also used to smoke up until around the time I became a vegetarian but now, the thought of drawing smoke into my lungs is as revolting to me as putting meat in my belly!

I had to do a fair amount of shopping around before I found a companion for Bubble. It was one of those periods when guinea pigs seemed to be in short supply. Though some people claim that this is always the case in the colder part of the year, I think this is a myth. Though I am certain that most behavioural and biological patterns of the domestic guinea pigs are very similar to their wild ancestors, in my experience, the matter of breeding times do not seem to come into that category. Of course it makes sense in the wild not to bring babies into the world during the colder months when there is a less abundant supply of food and it is harder to keep warm. However, this hardly applies when you have your own PP's to keep up the supplies and pay the heating bill!

I picked Squeak up from a pet shop in North London. She was about eight weeks old and from what I could glean from the books I had read that included sections on guinea pig breeds, she was classed as a Harlequin. This is a smooth coated guinea pig that has a coat of two colours. There will be and over all base one and the other will be in the shape of a spattering of a different colour, usually lighter. The effect is to look as though this colour has been applied by the flick of a paint brush.

The day I picked squeak up it felt as though it was one of the longest of my life. I had picked her up in the morning on my way to my first job site and then had another couple to visit during the rest of the day. This meant that Squeak had to put up with the noise and the jolting about in the small, hay filled box that the pet shop had supplied, which I had wedged very firmly in the passenger seat of my truck. It was bad for me too for I had to put up with the frustration of having to wait to make good on my promise to Bubble the night before.

"You'll feel much better with a little mate to play with while I am away at work all day and I do promise to double up the food supply," I had assured her, as I kissed the top of her head before putting her back down into her quarters. She was still a wee bit unsure about this kissing business. After all, the PP had a much larger mouth than hers and though his teeth were not as needle sharp as hers, there were a lot of them!

To some, the sight of a grown man holding a conversation with a wee small animal can be somewhat shocking. They may even regard it as demeaning that a human being should be so 'silly.' However, I have always 'Doolittled' and I had no intention of changing a lifetime's habit because of the hang-ups of other human beings. Besides, I had many years of being beastie bereft to catch up on!

I had spoken to many human beings in my life and heard them speaking to one another, so to speak, on the media. In the main, they made very little sense, or those that did were seldom listened to or taken what they said, taken seriously. Their talk had lead to many wars over religion, race, nationality, or any excuse to have a good old blood bath and keep the population figures down or satisfy that thing they call 'honour.' As for the other things they waffled on about, like sports, the arts, and what they owned and others didn't, boring, boring, boring. I think myself, and society is under less of a threat by my talking to animals than in my engaging in the many 'normal' activities of my kind! This is why, fifteen years after Bubble arrived, the Gurney-guinea pig debating society has expanded in direct ratio to the number of their kind that have come into my life!

If there ever had been any doubts in my mind about getting another guinea pig, Bubble would have disbursed them by the way she reacted when I put wee baby squeak into her quarters that evening. She had come to the front of her quarters in eager anticipation of the evenings grass or whatever other vegetable matter I had got for her. This time she was presented with one of her own kind, who immediately sought sanctuary under the hay. Bubble paused, peering up at me, then did a kind of double take, then turned and hastened after Squeak. There followed a great deal of purring and movement from beneath the hay and I left them to it while I went out to get the grass bag.

The sight that met my eyes when I returned was heart warming, to say the least. The pair of them were out on top of the hay and now Bubble was grooming Squeak around her head with her tongue. It was vigorous and enthusiastic and Squeak was responding by purring. She was crouching low, and still looked a little unsure of herself, but it was clear that she was no longer frightened.

By this time, of course, Bubble had become much more confident and I would watch her as she pottered about the room during the evenings. This night, the first with one of her own kind to play with, she did not venture out at all. This pleased me greatly for I liked the idea that she would no longer have to spend her days in loneliness.

About one week later, Bubble was dead and I was to shed the first of so many tears for the loss of a guinea pig.

Being a new and very conscientious owner, I was somewhat paranoid about the health of my new friends, so when I noticed a couple of bald patches behind Bubble's ears, when I was sitting with her on my lap, I became concerned. I had read that these animals could suffer from parasitic skin conditions, which if not treated could drag them down very quickly. This was wrong. Though the presence of parasites can lead to more serious conditions developing, it is certainly not a rapid process.

Little did I know at that time that all guinea pigs have these patches behind their ears to a lesser or greater degree. If I had sought the advice of a breeder or long term owner of guinea pigs they would immediately have put my mind at rest by pointing out that this was a natural phenomenon. However, I went to a vet, resplendent in her white coat and certificate of competency on her surgery wall and with the letters M.R.C.V.S. after her name! Mistake, big mistake and it was to cost Bubble her life!

"Oh yes," says white coat, confidently. "This is a minor parasitic condition and we can clear that up in no time with an anti flea powder." She then merrily spread a white powder all over Babble's coat because she said that it was important that the parasites were prevented from spreading.

I took Bubble home, and because I thought that it was possible that the parasite could be passed onto Squeak, I kept her on her own in the cage that I had used when I had first got her. The following morning, as soon as I opened the bathroom door a terrible odour hit me and there was Bubble, looking thoroughly miserable, fluid diarrhea pouring out of her. I cleaned her up as best I could and rushed her to a vet who was much closer to me than the one I had taken her to during my rounds on the previous day.

I told this vet exactly what the other one had done and was told to leave Bubble with him. I phoned the surgery as soon as I got home that evening only to be told that Bubble had died during the day and was asked if I wanted them to dispose of the body. In a daze, I told them yes and before I had replaced the receiver the tears were streaming down my cheeks. I sobbed like a child, sitting on the floor, my head in my hands and rocking too and fro. The last time I had felt such grief, cried as bitterly and felt so lost was when my father had died many years before.

To feel as much pain for the loss of a small animal as that which I had felt for the loss of my father is something that many people would not understand. However, I know one person would, that was my father himself. He was a wise man and he brought his children up to believe that human beings were not as special as they thought they were in the scheme of things, and that love of an animal was as valid as love for one of our own kind.

Though I didn't know at the time, the vet who had treated Bubble was entirely to blame for her premature death. This one, like many of her kind, had not the faintest idea of the behavioural patterns of a guinea pig. Putting flea powder on the coat of an animal that spends a great deal of it's time grooming itself, and whose gut flora is so delicately balanced as a guinea pig's is, was a recipe for disaster. Bubble, who up until the time she had been treated by a vet for a condition that wasn't suffering from, had been perfectly healthy, had simply ingested too much of the flea powder and had died of poisoning.

I had an e mail from an owner recently, who's vet wanted to use this kind of powder on her guinea pig. What made it even more appalling was the fact that this was a lactating mother with three babies suckling from her. Things have not improved in the fifteen years since Bubble was killed by the white coat!

The fact that this particular owner had more common sense than the many lettered professional no doubt saved the life of his guinea pig and her young. I warned him, as I warn all owners of guinea pigs, to keep as much distance between the average high street veterinary surgeon as possible, unless they knew of one who had a proven record of competence in the treatment of the species. As he asked if he could bring his guinea pig round to me for me to treat I readily agreed. Not at all to my surprise, as soon as I saw her I was able to tell the owner that the vet had also made a wrongful diagnosis. The hair loss that the vet had put down to parasites was nothing else but due to the very common hormonal imbalance that many pregnant sows suffering from when pregnant.

Even before Bubble's tragic death, I had it in mind to expand my family so by the end of that week I had two more guinea pigs and my local D.I.Y. store had my custom again for I had grand plans about improving the accommodation.

Katie was a tri-colour, 'dolly mixture,' which means that she was a very mixed, smooth coated breed. She had huge soulful eyes and her coat was black, brown and white. Pearl came from a local pet shop that didn't usually sell animals but the proprietor told me that this particular one was a reject from a breeder friend of his who showed his animals. She was a silver agouti but because the hair around her eyes was brighter that the rest of her coat, and she had a small heart shaped white patch in the middle of her back, she was not regarded as show quality.

To say that she was the breeder's loss and my gain would be a massive understatement. Seven years later when my third book, 'What's my guinea pig' came out, in which I was able to write about her death from old age, after a full and happy life with me, my description of her death was the cause of many kind compliments. The poignancy of her end made readers cry as much as I did at the time that I lost her.

My only regret was that I never bred from her for she was one of the most sweet natured little creatures that I have ever known, and I have met quite a few of them during the past fifteen years. It taught me a lesson, and though I still do not go in for a lot of guinea pig breeding, the premium on what space I have being for sick and unwanted guinea pigs, if there is one of those special ones then I will breed from it.

Not long after the arrival of Katie and Pearl I made a big mistake, one that is made by many new owners of guinea pigs. The fact that the R.S.P.C.A. books, until very recently, still recommend that what I did then is still a good idea, is a indictment of it's ignorance about just two of the animals that it is supposed to protect.

I went out and brought a rabbit to live with my guinea pigs!

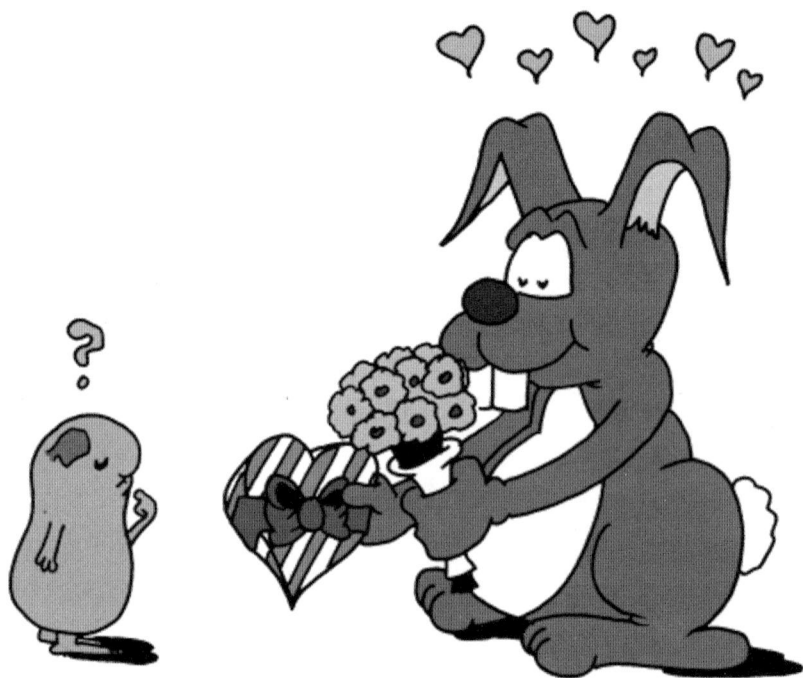

Chapter four.

Not a good idea.

Barnaby was a very handsome, medium sized rabbit but like many of his kind, very hyperactive and inclined to kick out with his powerful back legs. This is a very well known phenomenon that is the biggest danger to cohabiting guinea pigs, which can suffer serious and sometimes fatal damage when they are kicked by rabbits. If they are buck rabbits, then the proverbial rabbity randiness is also a hazard. No matter how cute and cuddly he may look, being mounted by one when you are a third or even less his size, is not a very pleasant or healthy experience.

Luckily, the then current guinea pigs, and all the subsequent ones that came to live with us during Barnaby's lifetime, all managed to adopt the 'hedgehog' method of defence against rabbit rape! They would immediately tuck their back and front legs in and bunch their bodies into a tight ball when Barnaby was on a high rut rampage. This meant that if Barnaby managed to get his front legs over the front of the guinea pig he couldn't engage the business end at the guinea pig's nether regions. So my guinea pigs managed to be shaken but ungoosed.

It was most frustrating for the poor lad but as it meant that my guinea pigs retained their virginity I compromised and never dragged him off the object of his passion. I figured that as I wouldn't be there all the time to do my U.S. cavalry bit it was best to allow my guinea pigs to rely their own anti seduction techniques! Now, of course, I am totally against rabbits and guinea pigs cohabiting.

Meanwhile, thoughts of procreation were stirring in my mind for Squeak. I just thought that as my mind was running along the lines of yet more expansion in the piggy population why not try some D.I.Y. or leastwise let Squeak try it.

I managed to borrow a handsome, black smooth coated boar and hoped that squeak would share my enthusiasm for this sleek, broad shouldered lad who had such a wonderful sheen on his coat.

"It's nookie time," I declared, as I put the box containing the boar down in the opposite corner to where the new enlarged quarters were. The girls didn't seem impressed and were more interested in the evening rations, which were duly served them. I made sure that the lad had a very generous helping as well, of course for he had work to do that evening so I wanted him well stoked up for the business in hand!

After I had fed and watered myself, had a nice soak in a bath, cleared a bit of space in the living room, leaving no area where they could enjoy a bit of privacy, I sat down in eager anticipation. I guess that all I needed as a dirty raincoat to complete the picture of a dirty old man with his eye to the bedroom door!

Though Squeak was the victim marked down for ravishment, I wasn't so silly to think that the boar would necessarily share my taste in sows! Besides, as he was destined for only one night of love, I thought that the very least I could do was to offer him some kind of choice.

Though Katie was only three and a half months old, she was of age, as it were, just. If I had taken the trouble to read up on the subject more thoroughly the first thing I would have learned was that sows were only fertile and fruity when they were in season, which occurs every fifteen to seventeen days. I thought it was the same kind of procedure that applies to my own kind. It was simply a matter of the business being done at any time during the cycle and that was it!

From the moment that I took Katie and Squeak from their quarters their differing personalities dictated the whole course of their actions. I set them down in the middle of the room and it was pretty clear that they had picked up the scent of the boar for they both stood stock still, looked in the direction of the box, raised their heads and sniffed the air interrogatively. Katie looked concerned and a little confused, then deciding to play it safe, trotted over to a corner of the room furthest from the box, where she sat down and waiting for Squeak to make her move. Her wait was a short one!

Tentatively, at first, Squeak moved towards the box, sniffing the air as she went, then increasing her pace she trotted right over to it, first scratched at it and then gave it a good nibble. She began to get excited, pawing at the box, purring and wriggling her rear end.

I went across and lifted the boar out and planted him on the floor in front of Squeak, who ran back a few paces and then I went back and sat down to watch the fun.

Squeak made her move, walking boldly up to the boar and gave him a quick sniff and then without more ado started to rub herself along side him, sensuously. She followed this up by turning up the volume of the purring, just to make sure that he got the message. She ended her dance of desire by turning her back on him and rubbing her bottom in his snout. Subtlety and decorum were not the kind of words that had any place at all in this little lady's language of love!

The boar's reactions to this offer of 'on a plate and gift wrapped nookie' were quick and decisive. He took to his heels and hid behind the box.

'Just my luck,' I thought. 'They've loaned me a gay guinea pig!'

The boar had obviously underestimated Squeak's determination to have her wicked way with him for she disappeared around the back of the box P.D. Q. There were the sounds of much frantic activity from behind the box, then he shot out from the other side of the box and ran across the room to a spot not far from where Katie was had been watching the proceedings, very warily. She tensed as he paused, one forepaw off the ground, head raised, sniffing the air about a foot away from her.

He obviously found whatever scent she was giving off as far more inviting than Squeak's had been for he began to purr and wriggle his backside in a most suggestive manner. There was definitely a lot of 'Well hello sweetie, where have you been all my life?' about it. Her response was to react in the same manner that he had when Squeak had made her move on him. She shot off to the right, heading in my direction with the boar in hot pursuit.

For the next couple of minutes I watched as the boar chased Katie, with Squeak following up in the rear before I decided to intervene. One thing was for sure, whatever else was happening, coition was not, and that was the object of the exercise. I simply lifted Katie up out of the chase, returned to my chair and sat her down on my lap.

The boar had shot away towards the box and hidden behind it again when I had scooped Katie up. Squeak, who had rushed in the opposite direction, was now doing a bit of head and snout grooming while she was catching her breath.

It wasn't long before the boar ventured out to see what had happened to the object of his passion, and finding her no where in sight, simply turned his attention upon Squeak. Whether this was because his engine was all fired up, resulting in an 'any port in a storm,' syndrome, or because he had suddenly seen her in a different light, I couldn't guess at. On the other hand, Squeak either decided to make him work for it or was surprised by is sudden rush upon her for a second chase around the living room ensued.

The chase didn't last long for quite unexpectedly Squeak suddenly stopped, turned and began to match him purr for purr, bottom bump to bottom bump. This time the boar got the picture and immediately began making mad passionate love to her, but to the wrong end! Squeak head butted in the belly a couple of times, twisted away from him, turned and crouched, splay legged, presenting him with her rear end. She didn't have to elaborate further for the lad jumped upon her and obliged her with great gusto. It was short, sharp and very vigorous, and afterwards he stuck his nose in her rear end as though checking to see that he had hit the target correctly.

I left the pair of them free ranging in the living room all night, just in case they needed to make sure with another session. If they did, they did so quietly for I slept soundly and awoke to find the pair of them in the small open fronted box that I had provided for them. I had put Katie into their proper quarters and blocked off the entrance in case he decided to have another go at her.

I took the boar back to the owner, thanking her for his services and informing her that I was pretty certain that he had done what was required of him. I promised to keep her informed about future events as a result of his night's toil.

My mother, sister and brother got the first indication of what was in store for them in the shape of a very 'prospective father' at the end of the telephone line the following evening. I gave them a blow by blow account of the deflowering of my little lady. I must say that they sounded very tolerant of my ranting and wished Squeak all the very best!

There wasn't a lot of in-depth information about what to expect throughout the course of Squeak's pregnancy in those days, apart from the fact that the first indication that a sow had clicked was an increase in her water intake about three weeks into her term. In the light of the fifteen years of experience of living with these creatures and going through many pregnancies, I know that this doesn't appear to happen in all cases. However, Squeak, bless her, made it easy for me by doing a text book job of the whole business, and did indeed start making more trips to the water bottle about three weeks after her night of delight.

As the weeks progressed, she began to swell out in the flanks and her appetite greatly increased. When the day came that I sat her on my lap, cupped my hands around her tummy and felt the first kick of a baby guinea pig, I think that I ascended to some kind of higher plane. Now, all this time and many pregnancies later, I still get that same kind of thrill when a feeling the stirring of new life in a pregnant sow.

When Squeak was about seven weeks into her term, my mother came down to stay with me for a week-end. I think she was checking things out to see how her 'little boy' was coping with his new family!

"Hm, kicking eh!," said my mother.

The pair of us were looking down at squeak who was lying on her side in the pen, rotund and very large, half mooned alongside Pearl. She had just moved her position slightly in response to a wave-like motion from inside her that was followed by what looked like a poking from inside, which I would have guessed a baby guinea pig's foot!

I glanced sideways at my mother, seventy five years of age, a mother of three herself, and caught the wisp of a smile of empathy with that small animal. She obviously knew just what Squeak was feeling, despite the many years since the time when she had gone through the experience.

"Did I kick like that?" I asked.

"Oh yes. Indeed, you did!" she replied with feeling.

I didn't know whether to apologize or to ask if my brother and sister were as active so I said nothing.

I am sure that by the conclusion of the week-end that she stayed with me my mother was very pleased with the turn of events in her son's life, and also convinced that this was no passing fad. She had seen me in love so many times but this time it was definitely for real. Neither she, nor my father had been hands on parents once we children had flown the nest, and in that way they brought their children up the way that most animals do, for that I shall always be grateful to them. We were taught to be self- sufficient, and were expected to cope with life as it came. However, I am equally certain that every time one of us stumbled along the way in life that they suffered the bruising as much as we did.

By eight weeks, Squeak was Mandolin shaped but though she looked so ungainly, she scurried about the pen with the same zest and energy as she had when she was a slim, lithe virgin!

During the last few days of her pregnancy my family had quite a few phone calls informing them, in high excitement, that she was about to give birth, only a few moments later to be phoned back and told that it had all been a false alarm. I kept mistaking her suddenly getting to her feet, going down into a kind of crouch position, which I presumed was stance for delivery time. It was, of course, nothing more than for the 'delivery' of pellets!

In the event, Squeak must have thought that she had had enough of me squatting down in front of her quarters and asking her, in a pleading tone, "come on, when are you going to do the business?" and decided to put me out of my agony. However, she had no intention of giving me a grandstand few of her littering down. I reckon that she must have waited until I had closed the door behind me on the due morning and thought to herself, "Well, that's him out of the way for the day. I'll get on with it now!"

Needless to say, when I arrived home each evening during those last few days of her pregnancy, I had been rushing into the living room, excited and hopeful. The evening of the morning of her 'performance' I stopped mid stride at the sight before, my excitement level going through the roof, my hope re-warded in abundance. There, behind the glass front of the pen were two ador-able baby guinea pigs, one ginger and white and the other black and white. It was almost as though she was presenting them to me with a 'Well, will these suit you, sir?' kind of air.

I fell to my knees in front of that little animal, mumbling over and over again, "you clever girl, you clever, clever little girl!" I don't think I had ever ex-perienced such utter joy and exhilaration in my life before and my eyes began to water. This time, the tears that were running down my cheeks were ones of deep gratitude at the wonder wrought in my home.

Phone calls were made all round to inform every one about this 'stupendous' event, which was followed by a large measure of scotch that evening to wet the baby's heads.

Though I didn't know it at the time, of course, the fact that she was already suckling her babies was clear evidence that she had littered down very early on in the day. Mother guinea pigs do not come into milk for between twelve and twenty- four hours after birth, and I believe it is the same for most human mothers. This isn't a problem for the young for they have sufficient nutrients stored within them to keep them going for twenty-four hours. However, I have seen many guinea pig mothers come into milk within six to eight hours and Squeak was obviously one of them.

The following five weeks of watching Squeak caring for her babies was a revelation to me. There is a combination of deep tenderness and business-like efficiency in the way that these animals get one with the vital business of nurturing. Every time I came into the room to see squeak, hunch backed and with that intense look in her eyes as she suckled her young, my heart was filled to bursting point. Little did I know that my mind was gathering material for a book I was to write twelve years later about the sex life of the guinea pig. I noticed that at the same time as the young were drinking their fill, Squeak would occasionally flip them over on their backs, or they would roll over, their mouths still firmly attached to her nipples. She would then set too and vigorously lick their genital area. Much later, I learned that this was what most mammals do to stimulate their young to defecate.

The ginger and white baby turned out to be a sow and the black and white was a boar. The sow's ears were basically pink but with a patch work of brown and white patches and as I thought that they looked a bit of a pickle that's what I named her, Pickle. As the boar was going to be taken by a friend of mine I didn't bother to name him.

Towards the end of five weeks, the babies went less and less to their mother and she soon began to push them away when they did so it was clear that her milk was beginning to dry up. Guinea pig usually lactate for up to six weeks but five is more usual in my experience.

The boy was definitely showing signs of sexual interest in both his sister and mother and the other sows in the pen so it was definitely time for him to move on. Though I knew that he was going to go to a good home, I felt a terrible wrench when I handed him over.

A few years later, after watching the magic of yet one more mother and her babies for the umpteenth time, I wrote the following few verses and they are dedicated to all mother guinea pigs.

WATCHING YOU WEANING.

Watching you weaning, from first suckling until 'time to go,'
With as much pride as I would if they were mine own begotten.
Watching you weaning, little bottoms wriggling to and fro,
As they drink deep, the darkness of your womb long forgotten.

Watching you weaning, cleaning, being proud of what you had done,
As they grew daily, drinking of you, playing tag, being girls and boys.
Watching you weaning, as they stole food from your mouth for fun,
Then sat on your head, and ran down your back. Pests? Oh no, Joys!

Watching you weaning, your gentle eyes, alert, loving, content,
Mirroring all that their happy little hearts felt for you.
Watching you weaning, meaning for you what pure happiness meant.
No code, no dog collard dogma, just something that you naturally do.

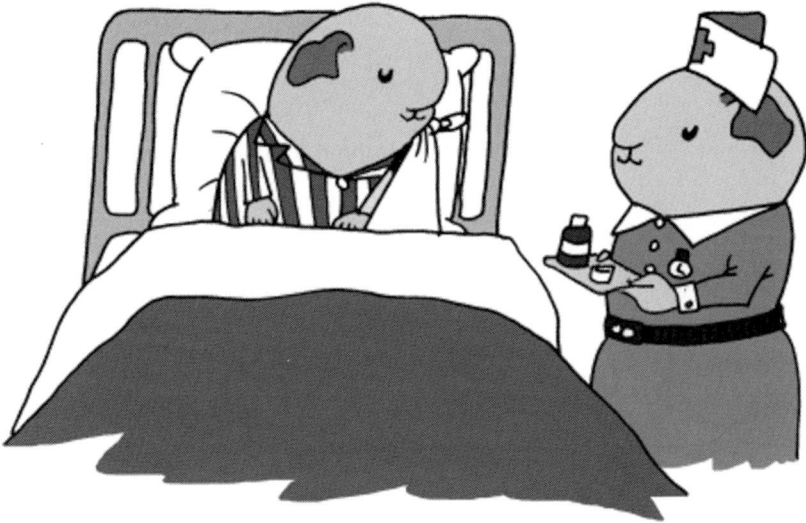

Chapter five.

The amazing lady.

It was the culmination of a series of events that had occurred during the course of a year after the birth of Squeak's babies that led me to seek out an amazing lady by the unusual name of Vedra Standley-Spatcher. In the main she was as concerned about the usual veterinary incompetence I was seeing and was just about to found the Cambridge Cavy Trust. However, it was the loss of Pauline, my sister, who died after many months of suffering from cancer of the colon that finally made me make this vital contact.

Katie, a wonderful tri-coloured sow, had developed a condition called Bumblefoot and after taking her to a local vet for treatment, she was dead within two days! Subsequently, I have owned and seen many other guinea pigs with this condition and in all that time no a single case has proved fatal. In essence, there is no cure for this condition but as it never leads to any other health problems, and is one that a guinea pig can learn to live with, I now never bother to treat one that is suffering from it.

In the light of fifteen years experience, I am convinced that the vet gave a contra indicated drug. For when I took Katie back the following day, when she had gone of her food, I saw another vet who immediately told me to stop giving the drug and gave me a powder, saying that it was vital that she was given it. The powder was a Pro biotic, something that is always used when an animal's gut flora has been damaged, particularly in cases where a drug has caused toxic effects. She didn't tell me of course, for the code of all sticking together, is as strong in the veterinary profession as in any other!

I had been increasingly voicing my doubts about the competency of veterinary surgeons when it came to the treatment of my animals. So when a friend saw an article in a news paper about a lady who was seeking to set up a State registered charity with the aim of trying to improve the veterinary care of guinea pigs I knew that I just had to get in touch with her. Little did I know, that as a direct result, a lifetime of programming to respect professional people was to be fundamentally altered!

For four long months my mother had nursed by sister to her inevitable death and the strain on her, in her mid seventies, had been painful to see. Two weeks after Pauline died, in November 1986, I decided to go up and meet Vedra and I insisted that my mother came with me. I knew that meeting someone new, and one who was obviously a great lover of animals, in a part of the country that I didn't think she had ever visited before, would be good therapy for her.

It was a lovely sunny, autumn Sunday morning and the drive from Luton took us about an hour and a half across Bedfordshire, Hertfordshire and up through Cambridgeshire, to the small village of Swavsey where Vedra lived.

When we arrived and Vedra met us at the garden gate, my first reaction was 'oh no!' for Vedra turned out to be strikingly like Pauline in looks and stature. However, it wasn't long before my mother was smiling, and chatting ten to the dozen, something I hadn't seen her do for a very long time indeed.

Vedra, who was very well aware of what my mother had been going through for the past few months, charmed her with a lap full of guinea pigs, and chatted away to her as though the pair of them had been friends for many years standing. This was the first of many examples I was to see of Vedra's wonderful way with people, which was as caring and considerate as her was her way with animals.

When I was shown around the purpose built block at the bottom of the garden, I knew right away that this lady really meant business. It was more like going into a mini hospital than a guinea pig refuge. There was even a functioning incubator with a tiny white guinea pig in a bed of hay in it.

One the walls were some horrific photographs of guinea pigs that had been misdiagnosed by professional veterinary surgeons. Many of these were of appalling skin conditions where the vets who had been treating them had been unable to differentiate between fungal and parasitic skin conditions. She told me that many guinea pigs died slow and painful deaths as a direct result of this professional incompetence when dealing with skin conditions. She added that be it fungal or parasitic, these skin conditions were very easy to treat if they were caught early enough and were correctly diagnosed from the start.

It was on this first visit that I learned of the appallingly restrictive laws governing the treatment of animals in this country that had handed the veterinary profession an unregulated monopoly of the veterinary care of animals. By unregulated, I mean total self regulation, which always amounts to the same thing. In essence, it always ends up with the protection of the provider of the service at the expense of the customers.

However, at the time, I guess I was a bit skeptical about some of what Vedra was telling me. In my long programmed mind I come to believe that it was gospel that all professional people were always to be trusted without question. These were the people to whom I had been taught to tug my forelock all my life. After all, they had had a university education, which meant that they had a higher ethical standard than mere oiks like myself! I had a great deal to learn! Oh, boy, a great deal to learn indeed! Now, fifteen years on, apart from a few exceptions, I expect to be cheated by, condescended to, and given a far lower standard of service from many professionals than I would get from the average Jill or Jo Bloggs! If anything, Vedra had been understating the level of incompetence that we had to tackle.

Even if veterinary surgeons in this country were adequately trained in the treatment of small animals, permitting them to have a monopoly, and then compounding the sin by allowing them total control of the complaints procedures against themselves, it would still be a recipe for a trade union rather than an animal protection measure.

We didn't leave until the evening and a date was set for my next visit over the next week-end for there was no doubt in my mind that I wanted to work with this woman and learn all that she could teach me. Though I lacked confidence in my ability to go back to school at this stage in my life, as it were, my conviction that my animals were not safe in the hands of professional veterinary surgeons was enough to spur me on. The greatest encouragement was, of course, the sight of Vedra's spectacular successes in cases where vets had written animals off as terminal.

So began my education, not only in the good husbandry and veterinary care of the animals I had come to love but in so many other spheres. That first week-end was the start of three years in which I spent nearly every week-end working and learning with Vedra.

The news of the Trust's existence was spreading even as I started that first week-end, so more and more people were bringing their guinea pig to the Trust. Before they were treated we got the owners to sign a form which stated that they were giving the guinea pig to the Trust but that they would get first refusal if and when it was decided to re-home it. This was, of course, a blatant legal device but both then and now, I firmly believe that the 1966 veterinary surgeons act, which was supposed to protect animals against incompetent practitioners was not thought even half way adequate. It would only have been justified if a proper complaints system, independent of the Royal College of Veterinary Surgeons was made statutory, and the training of veterinary surgeons in small animals medicines was radically improved.

There was another great advantage to working with Vedra and that was that it brought me into contact with people who had the same kind of values that I had when it came to my attitude towards animals. On more that one occasion, this aspect of the work brought me up sharp, to face my own preconceived ideas formed about certain people, putting them into stereotyped boxes. The most memorable lesson I learned occurred after I had been working with Vedra for about a couple of months when a farmer and his wife arrived clutching a box with an elderly ailing guinea pig sow in it. It was early afternoon and the farmer had phoned Vedra earlier on to ask if he could bring the guinea pig over.

Apparently, the couple had seen a T.V. programme in which Vedra had appeared a couple of months earlier, explaining why she had set up the Trust. They had driven all the way down from Norfolk in the hope that Vedra could do something for Rosie, their guinea pig. They told her that they were aware that at seven years of age, it was likely that Rosie was simply dying of old age, but they felt they had to give her the best chance possible and they believed Vedra was just that.

"I don't think you can save her," said the farmer, "but I know that if she has to go, her passing will be far more easy with you than with a vet."

It was clear that Rosie was suffering from a combination of pneumonia and renal failure and Vedra said that she had to agree with the farmer's prognosis but that she could certainly make Rosie more comfortable.

She put Rosie on some soft warm toweling, arranged like a small bed in the incubator, after she had given it a shot of something. Just before she pulled over the lid of the incubator, the farmer put his huge hand in and gently touched Rosie's head. It was tender moment, and clearly a goodbye gesture to an animal that was very dearly loved.

We all trooped back down to the bungalow where I made us all a cup of tea and we let the farmer and his wife talk.

"We got Rosie and her sister, Jenny, when they were about eight weeks old for our grandchildren but they lost interest in them quite quickly so we more or less took over the job of caring for them," they explained.

"We got very attached the them so we were quite happy to keep them our-selves" put in his wife. "Jenny' died when she was about four years of age and though we did think about it we never got round to getting another companion for Rosie. What we did do, was to bring her into the house and made a pen for her in the kitchen."

"For three years now," continued her husband. "We have been greeted by little Rosie's Squeaks each morning when we came down, asking for her break-fast and you can bet that she always got hers before we got ours."

They smiled when both Vedra and myself chorused that that was the way it was when you lived with guinea pigs. You don't train them, they train you!.

After having one last walk down to the block to have a look at Rosie, who was definitely looking as bit more comfortable, breathing much more easily, they left and drove back home after been assured by Veda that she would keep them informed.

Rosie died at about two o'clock the following morning, As usual, Vedra had been working in the block until about three in the morning.

"I checked her at about twenty passed twelve and she was definitely un-conscious then. Her breathing was shallow but not too laboured and I am sure that she didn't regain consciousness," Vedra, explained. "I checked her again, just before I turned in at about three and she had gone and I would have guessed been dead for about an hour.

The farmer and his wife arrived at about eleven the following day to pick Rosie up. They thanked Vedra and made a very generous donation to the Trust. I watched as they walked back down the garden path towards the gate with Vedra. I could clearly see from the shaking of the farmer's shoulders that he was weep-ing like a child. I hastily turned and busied myself in the task at hand of breaking down some bales of hay and back it up into sacks. I saw no point in both of us crying!

I have never gone along with the traditional image of country folk being kinder, gentler and more considerate that we urbanites for I have read about, and seen very many examples of callousness towards animals by country people and examples of gross arrogance towards town folk. That farmer taught me an important lesson. It was how wrong it was to label any individual by the bad behaviour of many of the peer group to which they belong.

"You're looking a bit pensive, something troubling you?" asked Vedra, when the pair of us were taking a mid-afternoon break that same day.

I grinned. "Oh now. I'm fine. Just learning a lot, and not only about guinea pigs."

I don't think I have ever been great shakes when it came to dealing with my own species but Vedra taught me how vital it was to be as concerned for them as I was about their animals.

They are your greatest ally," she explained, once. "It's their animal so they know it better than you ever will. Remember, the health history of a guinea pig is very important in helping you to make a correct diagnosis and it is the owner who knows it, so put them at their ease and get them talking. You can be puzzling over a symptom, which on it's own, isn't telling you much but sometimes an owner can tell you about an earlier symptom and eureka, what you're looking at suddenly makes sense."

Her basic outlook was that when you had a sick guinea pig to look at it wasn't alone, in most cases the owner was sick, sick with anxiety. You could help the owner, and yourself, by empowering them to take over the nursing of their animals themselves. It was far better for the animal to remain in the environment it was used to, which meant back home where it lived, usually with a companion. Only in cases where there was a possibility that it was carrying some kind of infectious disease, was it important to isolate a guinea pig.

"If ever I catch you doing what so many vets do, which is underestimating the knowledge that most owners have of their animals or their abilities to care for them when they are sick, then you'll feel my boot up your backside," she once warned.

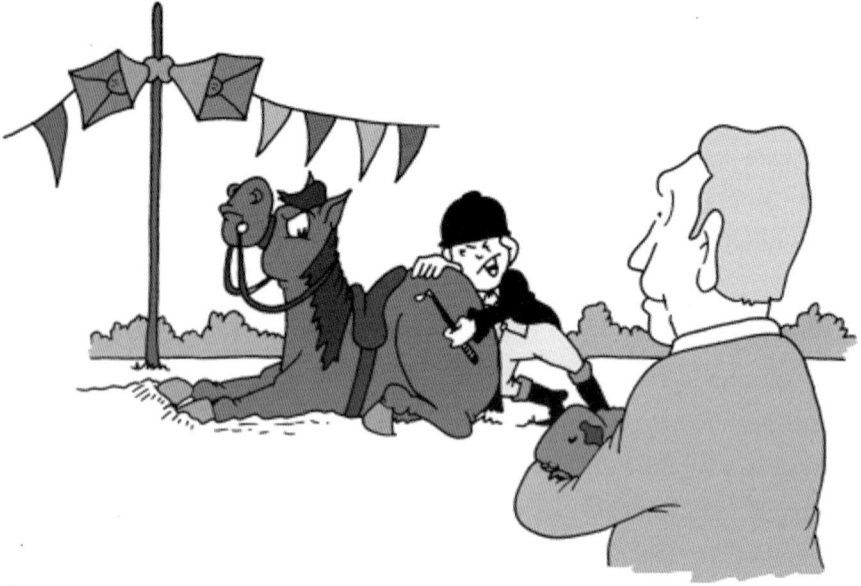

Chapter six.

G.O.S.H.

Even at the time of writing, some eleven years since I took the first guinea pigs up to visit the place, Gosh, is the expression I still want to make each Tuesday when I come away from there.

G.O.S.H. stands for Great Ormond Street children's hospital. The first time I visited there I was delivering building materials for a new block that was being put up. Chance would have it that during the month or so that I was regularly delivering these good I was to spend a Saturday at a gymkhana and it was the conjunction of these events that was to lead me to become Great Ormond Street's guinea pig man. It is a title of which I am very proud for to be associated with that wonderful place of the healing of children is a very great honor indeed.

How it came about was the result of my being in the right place at the right time.

As usual, things animal that had decided to mess up our plans that particular morning was a sow who had decided to litter down and then had problems delivering on her promise, so to speak.

We were about to leave for the gymkhana that was being held on land owned by a boarding stables a few miles away from the Trust. The proceeds from the event were going to be equally divided between the Disabled Rider's Association and the C.C.T., and we were going to set up a publicity stand there.

"You go ahead while I sort this little lady out," said Vedra. "I can't leave her, It's breach birth but it shouldn't take me long to sort her out, with a bit of luck and manipulation."

When I arrived at the site and explained the situation about the problem that had caused Vedra's delay, our hosts were very understanding.

"Tell me about it!" exclaimed the eldest daughter of the family who owned the stables, and who had been instrumental in getting the C.C.T. to be a joint beneficiary. Needless to say, Vedra had taken over this young lady's guinea from a vet, who though brilliant with horses, knew that guinea pigs squeaked out of one end and pooped out of the other but that was about the extent of his knowledge. However, unlike many of his kind, this vet was an honest one, admitted this deficiency and was only too willing to let an expert like Vedra do what he was unable to do.

"The day in this stables when everything goes according to plan, watch out for flying pigs," she said, with a grin.

She got someone to give me a hand unloading the trestle table, the two guinea pigs that I had brought along with me and all the publicity material. The guinea pigs in question were Simon and Garfunkel, two adorable Buff boars, They were brothers who were the best ambassadors we could have wished for. They had particularly gentle natures, loved being handle by humans, and all who met them fell under the spell of their pig soulful eyes.

It was a beautiful warm spring morning and the forecast for the rest of the day was clear skies and comfortable temperatures. I soon set up the stand and settled down in the sunshine with Simon on my lap. From where I was seated I would watch the arrival of the cars, most of which contained two or three children eager for the off and a horse box attached to the back.

Let me make it clear that though I adore all animals I have always been a bit nervous of horses. They are, in the main, very large and most that I have come across have seemed to be a tad skittish. I would imagine that a kick from one of them would bring tears to the eyes and a bruise or three!

I don't know how long these children, many of them very small indeed, had been working with these huge beasts but by their confidence and their control of them I would have guessed since they were in their cradles! Right from the initial backing of their mounts out of their horse boxes, with encouraging sounds and firm guidance, these little children were very much in control. Through the grooming and the putting on of the tack to actually getting astride them, these children had an air of authority that any army commander in the field would have admired. Later that day, I was to witness an amusing incident where this authority was very effectively challenged by a very crafty looking beast indeed but in the main, the children were very much in charge.

"Hello," piped a wee small voice from below and to the left of me, as I felt a touch on my knee.

Now I have always had a yen for blue eyed blonds and though this particular one was smaller and a lot younger than the usual ones that turned my head and made me make a fool of myself, she had it. She had it in abundance!

Her great big beautiful 'blues' looked up at me, and these, combined with the widest of smiles, conspired to have just the effect she was aiming for, complete compliance with her every command! She had obviously come into this world fully equipped with an ability to bend any man to her wishes and I was, of course a complete push over!

"And hello to you," I replied, lifting Simon and placing him closer to her on my knees. As this little charmer was clutching a fluffy tiger toy I felt that I should show her that I too had a 'toy' of my own, and a live on to boot. The little

46

boy in me had once again come surging to the surface and I felt that some showing off was in order. No matter how she tried, my dear old mother had never managed to cure me of this habit of mine!

The little girl's smile got even wider and she asked if she could stroke Simon. I said yes, told her his name and I asked her if she had any pets of her own.

She didn't reply, stroked Simon for a while then placed the tiger toy beside him, told me that I was to look after it, then turned and walked away to a small brick building that backed onto the road that I had come in on. I had been told that this was where we could get refreshment throughout the day. I presumed, correctly, as I was soon to discover, that this little girl was one of the grandchildren of the family who were holding the event.

"Hm, baby or perhaps I should say dolly sitting?" Vedra inquired, when she arrived about half an hour later. By this time I had acquired a rather immodest Barbie doll with a tattered mini skirt up where her bra should have been and with no knickers on. I had an 'heffalump' who's stuffing had gone awry, leaving it with a big bum and a somewhat reduced floppy trunk and a rather bedraggled Paddington bear with a wellie missing.

"I guess so," I replied, sheepishly. "There's this little minx who keeps bringing these----oh no, here she comes again." I had caught sight of her heading my way, this time clutching what looked like a knitted tortoise!

Vedra, grinned, and told me that she was indeed one of the family's grandchildren. I took the proffered tortoise, thanking young blue eyes for her largesse, then Vedra leaned down, scooped the little girl up into her arms and took her back to the refreshment building.

"Good result?" I asked, when Vedra returned, knowing by her manner that it had been.

"Yes. Three. Mum and babies doing fine," she said, her smile a mile wide.

We stood watching as more competitors and spectators arrived and I was gradually introduced to more of the family of the little girl as they busied themselves about the grounds. They were obviously a well organized bunch for they all seemed to have their allotted tasks and there was certainly a lot of them. Catering, checking entrance tickets, registering competitors for the various events, organizing the car parking and a myriad of other duties in order to get the show on the road.

Vedra had been around horses all her life and was an accomplished rider, and her knowledge of them was encyclopedic. At one stage in her life she had run a boarding stables in Wales where she had got to know a vet and his wife who not only taught her a lot about the veterinary care of horses but had become life long friends. This was a friendship that was to be very helpful when she decided to take on the business of improving the veterinary care of Guinea pigs. I was to learn a great deal about horses, their habits, and how to handle them by the end of the day.

"I can leave you in charge then?" asked Vedra, as she took off her coat and prepared to volunteer her services to the event organizers.

"Away you go and play and leave the important work to us. The Funkles and I have got it all buttoned up," I replied, ignoring the face she pulled at me.

This wasn't the first time that I had been in charge of the C.C.T. stand at a public event, and though initially I had been unsure of myself, I was becoming increasingly confident about my ability to sell the Trust. The fact that we always had a piggy or three on hand certainly made our message far easier to get across. Some of the animals that we took in had histories of neglect by owners, but more of them were the result of veterinary incompetence and we had some horrific photographs to illustrate this point. It was because of our determination to speak out against veterinary incompetence that we had such a strong support from long term owners of guinea pigs, many of whom were becoming increasingly disillusioned with the service provided by professional vets.

In retrospect, I think we were a kind of catalyst. Many of the people who visited our stand suspected that they had been ripped off by their vets or that their animals had suffered as a result of the incompetence of veterinary surgeons. However, they were too much in awe of the letters M.R.C.V.S, Member of the Royal College of Veterinary Surgeons, after the names of those who had treated their animals, to challenge them. I like to think that owners felt more confident to 'come out' as it were, when they became aware that there was a State registered charity, with a proven record of success, where the professionals had failed. They felt that they could stand up and be counted because we could also put them in touch with others who had been in the same boat.

To the right of where I sat there was a small paddock where the younger children were preparing their ponies and awaiting their turn to do their stuff. As the morning wore on and I watched these riders, it struck me just how good the cartoonist, Thewell was in portraying these kind of children and their world in his work. It was like watching a show of one of his cartoons. It was also here that I witnessed a pony getting the upper hand for a change!

A little girl, all dressed up in the pucker riding gear, complete with hard hat, from under which bright ginger hair curled out, having finished grooming her mount, decided to climb aboard it. Though it looked to my inexperienced eye that she had a firm hand on her pony, when she actually lifted her foot up to the stirrup, it managed to move just out of reach by stepping, ever so slightly sideways! There was definitely a kind of sneaky way in which this avoidance maneuver was carried out. She tired a second time, but again, when she lifted leg the pony adroitly repeated the move. The girl moved closer to the front of her pony then pulled his head around with her reins, and though I could not hear what she was saying I am certain that she was very firmly laying down the law to it.

The third time she tired to mount, her pony moved even further away. I saw the little girl clench a fist, then shrugging her shoulders, took something small and white from her jacket pocket and gave it to her pony, who immediately munched it down with great relish.

She moved back to its side, put her foot in the stirrup and the pony obligingly stood stock still, allowing her to climb into the saddle with ease. For me, the icing on the cake was the way that the pony turned its head just before it

49

moved off and looked back at me. Those big soulful eyes seemed to be saying to me, "She want's to ride me, she pays for it. That's the deal!"

Later, when Vedra passed by the stand to ask how things were going, I asked her what the magic white goodie was that the little girl had given her pony. I had expected to be told that it was some kind of specially formulated horsy treat.

"Oh, probably a Polo mint," she explained. "It's the best currency you can use when dealing with an upperty pony. Never fails."

By the middle of the afternoon people were making second visits to the stand, bringing along friends who had missed us, and it was the Funkels who were the big draw. They were handed round, hugged, their snouts kissed and in generally they were made a big fuss of. Some people just asked questions about the Trust while quite a few joined. Vedra took over for half an hour to give me a chance to stretch my legs and have a stroll round the grounds, which were now very busy indeed. The horses ranged from big sturdy Welsh cobs down through all shapes and sizes to the familiar Shetland ponies. The first were steady and passive, while the last were scatty and flamboyant.

I took over from Vedra, while she had to do her bit as the judge of the fancy dress parade, which was the last event of the day. There was the inevitable Calamity Jane, and Wild Bill Hickock, clowns, a red indian and a couple of cowboys, and even an assortment of riders in animals costumes, but sadly, none of them a guinea pig!

I had Simon and Garfunkel sitting comfortably on my lap and was feeding them an assortment of tit bits, feeling very content with myself. The sun was getting lower in the sky as the evening approached, and I felt a deep sense of satisfaction in the way that the day had panned out.

Some of the children were beginning to unsaddle their ponies and prepare for the journey home. They all looked amazingly bright and happy, and not at all tired after what must have been a very long and busy day for them. The thought came into my mind of how lovely it was that they had been raising money for the benefit of disabled people, many of whom where children like themselves and at the same time for the sick guinea pigs at the Trust. I guess it was a eureka moment again, when suddenly the idea popped into my mind that perhaps some of my healthy guinea pigs could visit the sick children at G. O.S.H. It turned out to be one of the best ideas that I have ever had n the whole of my life.

When I got home that evening, though I was absolutely tired out, I wrote a letter to the hospital, explaining who I was and asking if they thought that my idea of visiting guinea pigs would be something they would be interested in. I didn't really think that it would be favourable for though I had heard of the Pat dog organization that took dogs into hospitals, Guinea pigs! Would they! Could they!

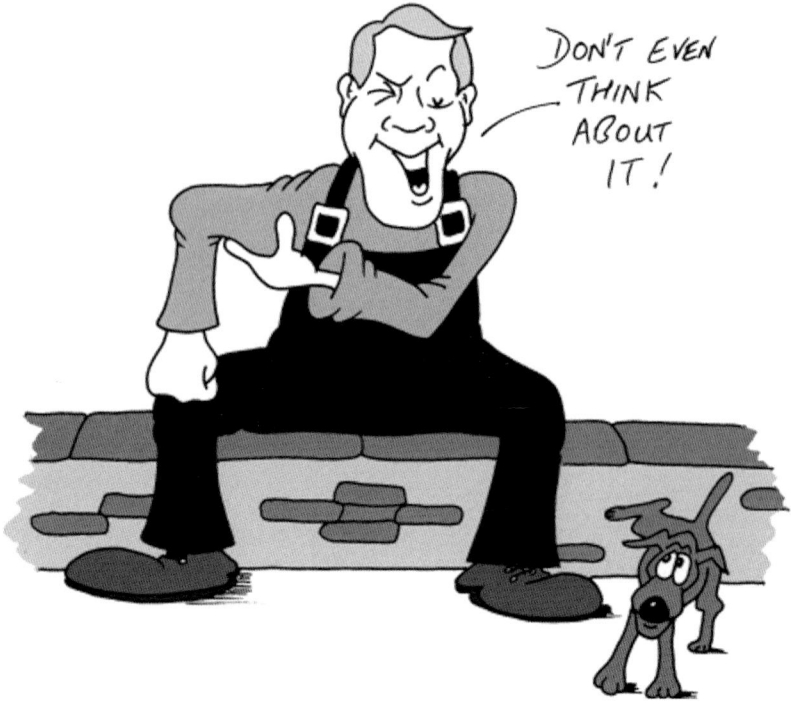

DON'T EVEN THINK ABOUT IT!

Chapter seven.

Boys and girls and broken bones.

I didn't have to wait long for a reply to my letter to the hospital. It was from a lady who ran what was called the play centre that I was soon to discover was a kind of nursery, come painting studio, come a wonderland of toys, come whatever the hospital thought would amuse or entertain it's patients.

The motto of the hospital is 'The child first, and always the child.' If anything sums of the ethos of that place then those simple words suit it to a T. This means that the fact that they are children is as a big a factor as that they are patients. For a child, being away from home is bad enough but the fact that they going into hospital must make it even more daunting.

Just walking into the entrance hall of the hospital, with it's wall decorated with familiar Disney and other cartoon characters, and the mood is set. There is a child sized London double decker bus that they can play in and video games dotted about here and there, and this is even before you get to the play centre, which is a riot of toys.

There is accommodation for parents so that they can be with their children so with mum, dad or both on hand the children can feel more at home.

The reply to my letter, which arrived about a week after the gymkhana, was friendly and positive. I was told that they thought it was a good idea and would I phone them for a chat and perhaps arrange for a day for a trial visit. I had a few days off work due to me so we fixed it for the following Wednesday.

The first visit was obviously a success as far as the hospital was concerned for we were warmly invited back again but it was definitely the beginning of a learning process. The arrangement of putting paper on a large table with the guinea pig on it in the middle and the children and their helpers sitting around was unsatisfactory for both piggies and people. The guinea pigs were nervous, tended to stay put and pee a lot, and the children of course, could handle them as much as they wanted to. After two or three visits, talking through the various things we tried each time, we settled upon a procedure, which in essence, we follow to this day.

Children were allowed, encouraged even, to hold a pet guinea pig if they settled one down with a towel spread on their laps. The golden rule was that they must never get up and walk around with them. Both the hospital and myself felt that for the sake of the contentment of the children, and the safety of the guinea pigs, this was a rule that had to be strictly adhered to. In the children's excitement there was always the danger that they would drop a guinea pig, and even from only a couple of feet up, it's still along way for one to fall and serious injury or even death could result. Apart from the danger to the guinea pig, the trauma to the child who was responsible, though not of course out of malice, was the last thing that it needed when in was in hospital.

We soon learned that very young children always had to be very closely supervised, and never left alone with a guinea pig. They tended to treat them like most children treat fluffy toys, and it amazing how many of them always seemed to want to poke the eyes. I suspect that with so many toys nowadays with buttons to push that they thought they were the guinea pig start buttons! Of course, once again, the actions of these very young children were not deliberately malicious, and because of the vigilance of the staff and myself not a single guinea pig has suffered any harm in all the time we have been visiting.

The biggest problem was the journey right across the busiest part of London from SW8 to WC1, where the hospital was situated. Even though I was traveling after the rush hour the drive was not pleasant and I could never predict how long it would take me. Parking was a pain, and though the hospital offered to pay for me to park in a nearby commercial car park, I was not at all happy about it. The journey by tube, with just a couple of changes en-route, would not take long but the problem was how to carry five guinea pigs with me. By car, I simply put them in some carrier boxes and put them on the back seat.

Vedra and a friend of hers, who happened to be a skilled coach builder by trade, came up with the ideal solution. Within a couple of weeks of putting my problem to them they had designed and made a long narrow plywood box with a hinged lid and a handle on the top, wire mesh down one side and six compartment in it. The only problem was that with a full load of guinea pigs in it, it was a wee bit on the heavy side. I had to consider that there was a good fifteen minute walk from my home to the tube station and a ten minute one from Russell square to the hospital. Add to this the stairs and escalators that had to be negotiated on the journey, and it was obviously that it would be quite a trial of strength. The answer was to put a couple of wheels on one end of the box and a flip up handle at the other and I could trail it along behind me.

Very early on I got into the habit of putting on a G.O.S.H. plastic apron as soon as I arrived at the hospital for, as I explained to so many people who asked about it, I was liable to be leaked upon at some stage during my visit. Being a bit of a ham and a show off, I soon began putting the apron on before I left home and this is what I do now, eleven years later. The guineas were a great conversation starter on the journey to G.O.S.H., and wearing that apron drew even more attention to us. Many a morning we have managed to turn some grim faced commuters on their daily grind to work into happy smiling individuals as they began to talk about guinea pigs they had owned in their youth or of their current pets.

In good weather the play centre had access to an open air play area with fixed, child sized model cars, a train and some climbing frames. In one corner of this areas lived Flopsy, The G.O.S.H resident rabbit. Though he had his own elaborate quarters, he had the freedom to roam the whole of the play area. At first I was a little concerned about this for with so many children running about, allied to the fact that he was no spring chicken, I thought he was very vulnerable. However, as proved by his great age, he had survived very well indeed with all these hazards and I was soon to learn that he was a very wise old cove when it came to the business of seeking his own space when he had had enough of the children. He knew all the spaces where he could seek sanctuary from those small grasping hands, and it didn't necessarily mean that he had to hide. More often than not you could find him under the train or one of the cars, right in the centre, tantalizingly in full view of the children but just out of their reach.

Flopsy was retired about eighteen months after we began visiting G.O.S.H. but went on to live out a further year at an animal refuge.

The media interest in the Trust began to include myself, and Celia Haddon, a journalist for a national newspaper asked if she could write an article about me and my involvement with the Trust and the hospital. This was picked up by someone at the B.B.C's T.V. Blue Peter programme, and I was asked if I would be interested to be a guest on it and bring along some of my guinea pigs. I readily agreed, for two reasons. I was becoming convinced that those responsible for the regulation of the veterinary profession would not budge an inch. However, this profession was, and still is, very image conscious and as the media was so important in maintaining their public image, then it would be wise of me to cultivate it myself.

The second reason, was that the more I visited G.O.S.H. the more enamoured I became of the place. It was the antidote to that strong streak of misanthropy in me, which though it had stood me in good stead down the years in dealing with my own species, it could be dangerously labeling of all of their kind. I guess I thought that the more publicity I could bring to that place then it would give human beings a better press. I wanted the whole damn world to know more about that wonderful place.

A date was set for the Blue Peter appearance and I was looking forward to it, for I would be doing what I enjoyed the most, showing of my wonderful wee beasties. However, fate decided that it was time to finger me, in the shape of a very nasty accident only a week before we were due to appear on the programme.

The truck that I drove had HiHab crane on the back of it, just behind the cab with which I hoisted off the heavier loads when I was on site. Having operated these cranes on various types of trucks for the previous twenty years, I was very experienced and should have known better than to make the fundamental mistake that I made on the day of my accident.

I had passed the two lifting straps under the last pallet of breeze blocks that had to be delivered, hooked them up to the jib of the HiHab and all I had to do was climb down the side of the truck to work the controls from the ground. Note, climb down, not jump down. Jumping down was what young inexperienced beginners did and were all warned was a definite no-no in the safety instruction that we all had to be familiar with when we operated HiHabs!

I jumped, caught my left foot in one of the slack lifting straps. This had the same effect as though someone had just grabbed my ankle and held it firm, launching out into the air at about five feet above the ground. This, my first attempt at unpowered solo flight was lousy from start to finish. The take-of was iffy, and I decided that I had the gliding qualities of the average house brick, the landing was catastrophic! I had plunged outwards and down, my momentum greatly increased by the sudden tug on my left ankle. At the last split second I flung my right arm outwards to break my fall.

The first thing I noticed as I slammed down hard on the hard on the road surface were my glasses sliding away from me towards the curb opposite. Despite the sever winding I do remember thinking, "Good, at least I haven't broken my glasses."

I felt a bit nauseous and was very unsteady but I managed to stand up. Once I was upright, I looked down at my right arm and to my astonishment it was swinging, pendulum-like, from the right elbow.

"It shouldn't be doing that," I thought, as I reached down with my left hand, caught hold of my right and lifted it across my chest and held it there.

I few days later, my boss told me that the chap working on the site said that as I walked round to the pavement I said, in a quiet, matter of fact way, "I think I've broken my arm, mate." He said that though I looked pretty shaky, I seemed pretty calm about it and for a second he thought I as joking. It was only when I came level with him that he could clearly see the jagged bones, which I was later to learn were the shattered ends of both my Ulna and Radius bones, that he really believed me. I told my boss that if ever he came across that chap again to thank him from the very bottom of my heart for not informing me of those bones!

The chap sat me down on a low garden wall, recovered my glasses and called a couple of his mate to stay with me while he went off to phone for an ambulance. The pain was now intense, though, strange as it may seem, I had hardly been aware of it until I sat down. A small dog came up to me from a nearby garden and began to sniff round my legs, speculatively!

Now let me make this clear right from the beginning, Peter Gurney is not the stuff that martyrs are made of but there is a definitely a lot of the grin and bare it Englishman in my make up. The ethos of not making a fuss over, say, a thousand pound bomb falling on your head, and the like, must have been well installed in my psyche by growing up during the dark days of the second world war. Therefore, the notion of making a fuss of such a 'minor' detail such as an arm that looked as though it was hanging on by a thread, and was likely to fall off completely at any second, didn't really enter my mind! However, though the old upper lip trembled not, I certainly felt the needed to a rabid bowel movement, and somewhere at the back of my mind I badly wanted my mum to come along and kiss it all better!

"Now you wouldn't cock your leg up at an injured man, would you?" I hissed through clenched teeth. The dog obligingly moved of and went about its business, so I remained dry legged.

So ingrained in me is the notion of not making a fuss that I felt more embarrassed that I had caused so much disruption to the working day of those about me and those back at the depot, than concerned about the condition I was in. Work at the site had come to standstill and my workload for the rest of the day would have to be shared out between my fellow drivers. I was certainly concerned about my wee beasties back home. To have another living, breathing creature dependent upon me was a bit of a novelty for I had been only responsible for myself for the past twenty five years.

The ambulance arrived in about ten minutes and I was rushed of to Ealing hospital, about a mile away. After being examined, the first question I was asked was when had I last eaten. Normally, I would have waited till much later during the day for my first break but on that particular day, digging it's finger in once more, had seen to it that I had had it early on. I knew that I had a busy day ahead of me so I thought that it would be easier if I had an early break and then I would work on right through until I had finished all my drops.

As I had eaten of course, this meant that it was not until that evening that it would not be safe for me to undergo a general anaesthetic for the initial surgical work to be done on my arm.

My boss had phoned, wishing me well and to tell me that arrangements had been put in hand for one of my work mates to call on a friend who had a spare key to my flat so he could let him in to feed the wee ones. He phoned me later that evening, just before I was due to be wheeled down to the operating theatre. He told me the guineas were fine and my friend and his wife would take over the cleaning and care of them for as long as it was necessary and that I was not to worry about them. The relief I felt at this news was immense, and they wheeled a much happier man down to the theatre than the one that had been brought into the hospital

I was allowed to go home at the week-end but had to be back at the hospital for the major repair job on my arm by the following Tuesday. I could hear the squeaks of greeting as I put the key in my front door that Saturday morning and it was the kind of welcome home that I had not known for a very long time. My heart warmed to them and each was hugged and told how much it was missed.

Later that day, someone from the Blue Peter programme phoned and when I told them what had happened they said if it was still O.K. with me could they still at least borrow some of my guinea pigs and particularly Mr Chipper. He was a beautiful tri-coloured sheltie that I had promised to bring with me. I readily agreed and we made arrangements for him and the guinea pigs to be picked up from my friend's home on the morning that the programme was due to go out.

Knowing that the care of my animals was in hand and that Chipper would still have his debut on T.V., I was keen to get back to the hospital and get the main operation over and done with.

The surgeon who worked on my arm told me that it had been a long and complicated operation for I had managed to make a kind of Humpty-Dumpty kind of job out of my elbow.

Myself and a couple of nurses managed to catch Chipper and the other's debut and all agreed that Chipper stole it! The presenters of the show were kind enough to wish me well and hoped that I would soon be back home again.

Little did I know that falling off that truck was to prove yet another "best thing' that had happened to me in my life. Because of the extensive damage done to my elbow, it was to be a long job and I was to undergo several other operations over the course of the next few months. I was warned that there was very little likelihood of my ever being able to drive a truck again but that I would certainly have enough strength in the arm to drive a car.

The really good news was that as the accident happened at work it was classed as an industrial injury so I was entitled to full pay. I had never griped at having to pay National Insurance for I have always believed that it was a good system that those who worked for a living should be properly provided for if they could not longer work because of injuries or illness. Of course, I never thought that I would ever have to claim off the system. I, like most of us, think that these kind of things only happen to other people!

What this all amounted to was that as soon as the plaster was off my arm and I had enough strength in it, I was able to drive up to the Trust. I always look upon this period at the real start to my training and the study of veterinary care of guinea pigs. It simply meant that I was able to work and study full time.

Simply watching Vedra work was an education in itself, and the light work that I could do was just the kind of thing that my surgeon had advised me to do as physiotherapy.

It was at about this time that I began to establish the G.O.S.H. visits on a regular weekly basis. . It wasn't long before I was made to realize that the therapy that myself and the wee ones were giving to the children could be a two way affair. The first clear instance of this came from a little boy who had been flown over from Northern Ireland.

This must have been about three or four months after the accident and I was still carrying around some screws and pins in my arm which, at times, caused a great deal of pain as the healing process continued. I was beginning to winge a bit about both the pain and the trips back to the hospital.

The little boy, who must have been about twelve, was minus a leg from the knee down, and one arm from the elbow. I presumed that it was as a result of the troubles for I was sure by the dressings on his stumps that the loss of these limbs were recent and it wasn't birth deformity. I never ask a child or the staff why the children are in the hospital as right from the start I made it a self imposed policy not to inquire as to why the children were there. One, it was none of my business and two, some of the injuries and illnesses that they were suffering from could have been caused by some traumatic event that they didn't want to be reminded of.

The first time I visited this little boy he was obviously still in a lot of pain for he was wincing quite a lot as he played with Chipper. I was sure that his pain was worse than mine, he was a long way from home and confined to a hospital bed but his zest and enthusiasm for the guineas was a joy to see. He asked many questions, and his constant laughter was just the kind of medicine that I needed to make me get a proper handle on things.

As I walked out of the main hospital entrance I heard little voice, saying, mockingly, "Gurney you are nothing but a wimp, a big girl's blouse." I even looked forward to my next week's visit to the boy for another hefty dose of that medicine he had administered to me. It was to be the first of many incidents I have seen of children simply getting on with it, no matter how bad the illness or injury.

It was about this time that my 'criminal' activities began to expand. Because of the increasing coverage in the media about the trust and the rapidly expanding membership of it, victims of veterinary incompetence and indifference, were becoming more and more aware that there was an alternative. London is a huge catchment area and as I was the only one living there at that time who had some training at the Trust, our London supporters all came to me.

I shall never forget the first really bad case of a guinea pig that had been misdiagnosed as having a parasitic skin problem when in reality it was a fungal one. His name was Mr Scruff, a tri-coloured Aby boar. Joan, his owner, was at her wits end and very distressed as her vet had suggested that after three months unsuccessful treatment, during which time Scruff's condition had worsened, that it was time to consider having him put down.

He had been brought to me on a Monday and the first thing I did was to phone Vedra, tell her what the symptoms were and ask if I could bring him up for treatment.

"Bring him up when you come this week-end but start the course of treatment yourself. You've seen me do it here enough times and helped with it so it's about time you did one yourself," she said, batting the ball firmly back into my court. The 'Oracle' had spoken so there was nothing to do but take on the task of taking on the responsibility of curing Mr Scruff myself. It wasn't only the suffering of the animal that made me take this responsibility so seriously, it was also my deep concern for Joan, who clearly loved him in the same way as I loved my own animals.

Within two weeks I was able to hand Mr Scruff back to Joan, well on the road to recovery by following the shampooing and dipping regime that I had learned while working with Vedra. I think it must have been one of the proudest moments of my life and Joan overwhelmed me with her gratitude.

I had done in two weeks what a fully qualified veterinary surgeon had failed to do in three months and in this, and subsequently many other cases, saved the guinea pig from unnecessary euthanasia. Mr Scruff was the first of hundreds of guinea pigs that I have treated illegally but I am proud of the fact.

Within a couple of years I would to come up with an alternative way of treating these skin conditions and it was the old 'necessity being the mother of invention' syndrome that inspired me. Most of the medicines that were required could only be acquired from a vet. As by this time I had completely lost confidence in the ability of the average vet to correctly diagnose skin conditions in guinea pig, this meant that even though they had a strangle-hold on the medicines they were unlikely to prescribe the correct ones.

I may have lacked five years training at a veterinary college but the one great advantage I was about to benefit from was the large number of guinea pigs that were to come under my care for my refuge for guinea pigs was about to come into being.

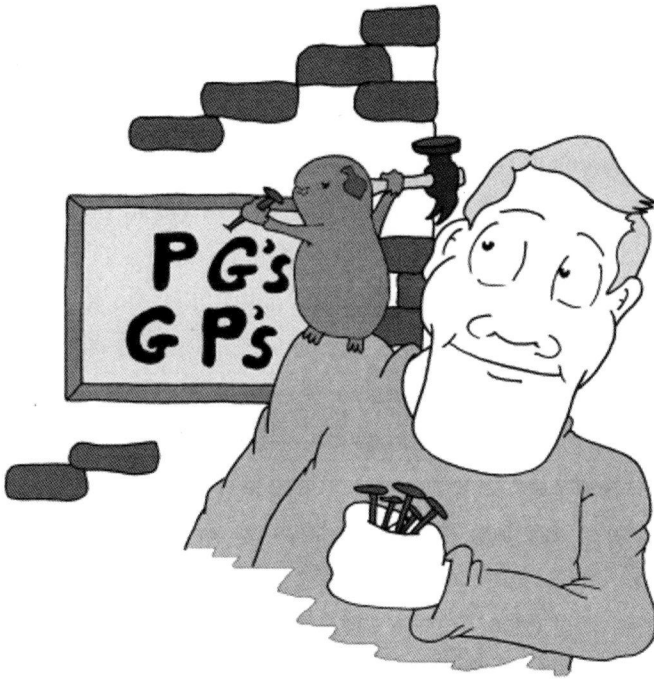

Chapter eight.

A year of firsts.

That my initials should be the same as those for guinea pigs, only in reverse, seems to me to have a whiff of destiny about it, and it didn't take me long to think up just the right name for my refuge, PG's GPs.

My refuge was nothing more than my home and I simply got some cards printed up and let it evolve naturally. As I was more interested in veterinary refugees than in unwanted guinea pigs, most that came to me were by word or mouth or via the Trust.

The services of PG'S GPs were to be required very desperately within a couple of weeks of it being established. A hundred and twenty guinea pigs, forty of which were pregnant sows, suddenly needed re-homing. These were from a young new breeder who had managed to get right out of her depth. Her breeding programme had gone totally out of control and she was not coping with either housing, husbandry or basic veterinary care of these animals. A great deal of the stock had been over medicated. The owner had not only made a habit of putting additives in the drinking water bottles but had been working on the principle that if the manufacturer of these products recommended, say 2ml per lire of water then four or five would do the stock even more good. As this had been gong on for quite a considerably length of time, it had caused renal and liver problems in some of the older stock.

By the time the rescue mission was over I had gained much valuable experience but when it begun I had another lesson in the way yet another public institution operates that did not impress me one little bit. This was the R.S.P.C. A., the premier charity set up to prevent cruelty to animals in the U.K.

The scenario was this. We had to pick up all this stock one week-end and transfer them to a rabbit and guinea pig refuge based near Heathrow and run by some friends of mine, Teresa and Colin Carter who had kindly agreed to take them all on. This would be a temporary arrangement until new homes could be found for the majority of the stock.

Needless to say, with such a huge influx of animals there was no way that they had sufficient pens or hutches to hold them all so a lot of phoning of friends and animals welfare organizations had to be done. All, with one exception, helped us or put us in touch with people who could. The exception was the R.S.P.C.A., [which was totally negative to our request.] This was in 1991, and subsequent experience of dealing with this organization has lead me, and many other people involved in animals welfare, to the belief that this is the last organization that we would go to seek help from if animals were being subjected to cruelty or needed shelter. We have come to the conclusion that unless there is a photo opportunity or they can prance about in front of T.V. cameras in the many misleading portrayals of veterinary care in this country, then forget it. At least this experience has taught us what animal charities can be relied upon to come up with the goods when the chips are down. One was the brilliant Animal Samaritans organization, which were a great help in

64

supplying hutches and names of people who would not only supply some but also deliver them. Between them we managed to get together all the accommodation that we required. By Saturday morning, after the Carters had worked throughout the night, their garden and house was full of pens, cages and hutches ready to house the refugees.

It was summertime and the weather was fine so most of the housing was arranged out in the garden. I went over on the Saturday afternoon with my veterinary hat on to give the stock a thorough check over and sort out those that needed treatment. Vedra had volunteered to treat the more serious cases and had put out feelers to the members of the Trust to find homes for are much of the healthy stock as possible.

At that time, Ben, an adorable bundle of fun, a tri-coloured peruvian with lots of other breeds in his lineage, was boarding with me while his owners were on holiday. He had been brought to me about a year earlier as his owner was not satisfied with the treatment that he was receiving from her vet. It took me a couple of weeks to undo the damage done by the vet and tackle the real problem he was suffering from and during the time that he stayed with me I got to know and become very fond of him.

Not only was there something particularly endearing about shaggy 'Bad hair day" looks, he was also a very laid-back dude and we soon became great buddies.

As soon as I arrived at the Carters, I put Ben in a pen on the lawn and settled down on a stool and began the veterinary check ups.

Many of the guinea pigs I examined could be treated by Teresa and Colin but a few of them only I could treat because by that time I had been trained to do the necessary dental work by Vedra without the use of anaesthetics. Even now, eleven years after the technique was perfected by Vedra, only a handful of vets have bothered to learn it. This results in the unnecessary deaths of hundreds of guinea pigs that are too weak to survive the anaesthetic that is required to carry out the outdated techniques that profession vets have been trained in.

As these cases would have to be taken home with me, because the work has to be carried out under a proper medical magnifying light, they had to be caged up separately, along with the cases for the Trust. The latter I would be taking up for Vedra to deal with on the following Monday.

Upon reflection, it is a sad indictment of the way English law works that these people, myself and Vedra, were all committing criminal offenses under the 1966 veterinary surgeons act by treating these animals and in many cases saving their lives. The law, and the authorities would have supported the status quo. I say again, and I shall continue to say it, methinks the law Hee-haws mightily. The older I get, the louder I get, and the more it grates on my nerves and the more contempt I have for the law makers and those that lobby to get laws onto the statute books to enhance their monopolies.

After a lunch break Teresa put what I thought was Ben into my lap.

"What do you reckon, A basket case, eh?, she asked.

"Hm, not a lot of hope for him. Have you got a hammer handy we'll put him out of his misery," I replied, solemnly, genuflecting and humming Abide with me.

"Look again," insisted Teresa.

I did as I was bidden, picking him up nose nuzzling him then said that after all that perhaps we could postpone the sentence for a while.

"Look over there," said Tereasa, pointing to Ben's pen. Once more I did as I was bidden and there in the pen was Ben, busily munching grass.

"Then who's this?" I asked, looking at the doppelganger of him sitting in my lap.

"One of the refugees," relied, Teresa.

"Tell me, tell me, tell me, that he's not been offered a home. Please," I pleaded.

"Nope, want him?"

"Want him! I'll fight any man in the house who dares dispute my claim to him," I declared, hugging my new acquisition tight to my chest.

I named him Fred and he became the first of a long line of free ranging guinea pigs. I'm not quite sure why I decided to make him go free range. Perhaps it was because I thought that I had my quota of boars, two, Chipper and Chester, and didn't want to fit out another pen. Looking at my wall to wall guineas now, having only two boars would make me feel that I was almost beastie bereft!

Having a free range guinea pig isn't something I would recommend to a family for the risk of it being trod on, kicked or getting itself terminally squashed in a closing door would be far too great. Fred was to be my 'guinea pig' in how to live with a free ranger.

After kicking poor old Fred a couple of times, and feeling very guilty about it, I decided to adopt a policy of 'running in' free rangers right from the start. It seemed to me that it was my responsibility to make an animal understand that it now lived with a great big clumping human being and it had to be trained to be 'flat-wise.' I developed a foot stamping technique which I describe in more detail in the Chapter about my free rangers.

Guinea pigs are far brighter than most vets give them credit for and Fred was no exception for he soon got the picture. My feet were just another hazard, like any other that guinea pigs have to put up with and he learned to live with them.

As with Chipper and to a lesser extent with Chester, I was being made aware that boars seemed to be a little more adventurous than the sows and settled down far more quickly with their human hosts. This certainly didn't mean that I valued the sows less but just recognized that I had to work harder with them to gain their trust.

By this time I had been living with guinea pigs for three years and learned that the 'getting to know you' part of the equation of life with them would always be challenging. Like all relationships, they had to be work on and as no two guinea pigs are the same you had to vary the way you got to know one another.

One of the top veterinary surgeons in this country with a column in a national news paper put six animals in order of preference that make good pets.

The last was the guinea pig, which he claimed was the least rewarding as they were very bovine and were the least active. This, of course, didn't come as any surprise to me. Sluggish, dull, stupid is the dictionary definition of bovine. Stupid is definitely a very accurate definition of this many lettered but little brained member of the R.C.V.S. Guinea pigs are the very antithesis of those three words and only a veterinary surgeon with the 'benefit' of five year training in one of our brilliant veterinary colleges could get it so wrong.

By the time Fred arrived I had already taken steps to make all telephone lines, speaker wires and electric leads inaccessible to the nibbling test, as giving my penned guinea pigs free range sessions during the evenings had become an established routine. I learned the hard way all about the delights of having my telephone and stereo system put out of action by those sharp incisor teeth! This experience gave me a running start when it came to having a full time free ranger running about my flat.

What I found so endearing about Fred was his increasing confidence to explore the felt within a very short space of time. At first, he stayed pretty much in the open fronted quarters that I had made for him in my kitchen but within a week he could be found in any room, including down the hallway into my bathroom.

Fred was about three years of age so was in his prime. Needless to say he took a very great interest in the sow pen. He spent a great deal of his time with his nose pressed up against the glass front of the pen like a little boy looking in a shop window at Christmas time, drooling over the goodies on display. There were times when a sow that was in season would hook her forepaws over the top of the glass and wriggle her hips at him. They still do this now to my free rangers and I have not yet figured out if this a deliberate tease or an open invitation! It certainly fires the boys up and poor old Fred used stand up on his rear legs, pawing at the glass, nose nuzzle and get in a high old state.

It was not till the end of the year, by which time all the refugee mothers had littered down and their young ones and been weaned, that we managed to re-home all the guineas that Teresa and Colin took in. All in all, we felt that we had every reason to congratulate ourselves but we all felt that we were merely paying off the bill that we all owe to these animals for bringing such pleasure into our lives.

Christmas came and went, and by spring 1991 yet another extension had been added to the sow pen and a tiered section had been added to house what I had begun to call my 'Kitchen cavies.' In April, almost a year to the day when I had broken my arm, I had another first, and one that I sincerely hope that I should never repeat.

I had been working very hard underneath my car one Sunday morning and by the afternoon I felt pretty whacked. Later in the day I noticed some blood in my urine and presumed that it could have been caused by my straining myself while I had been working. I should have known better and taken myself down to the hospital, when by the early evening the bleeding seemed worse.

Apart from feeling tired, which I put it down to the hard work I had been doing, I felt fine but before I turned in I resolved to go to the doctor first thing in the morning.

I had only been in bed for about a quarter of an hour when I began to feel a crippling pain low down on the left side of my back. I felt weak and my temperature began to rise, so I knew that I was in trouble and immediately phoned for an ambulance. I wanted to phone Vedra and my brother but I only managed to contact Vedra, by which time I was literally on my hand and knees in agony. She promised to phone my brother, asked me for the address of the friends who kept my spare keys, and assured me that the wee ones would be taken care of if I had to be in hospital for any length of time.

To this day, I still do not know how I managed to crawl to the front door and slip the latch so that the ambulance crew could get into me. As for the time it took them to reach me, I think that the pain blotted out all sensation of time and it could have been ten minutes or an hour. All I remember was that it was cold, or I felt cold, as they carried me down two flights of stairs in a kind of carrying chair, and very sick indeed.

There is no doubt in my mind that the night staff at St Thomas' hospital were some kind of aberration from the norm for when I consider the wonderful care and expertise I received at this hospital after that first night there can be no other explanation. I was give a brief examination, then shunted off into a small cubical with a trolley in it to lie on and left alone and not visited once throughout the night. During most of the night I was writhing in agony on the floor or trying to find a position to lie in on the trolley, which would ease the pain. I am certain that I was not a silent sufferer but not once did anyone come and check on me.

Much to my relief, at about seven in the morning a doctor arrived, gave me another brief examination and gave me a pain killer which kicked in very quickly and was powerful enough to knock out the pain completely. I still cannot understand why this was not done the night before. Friends of mine in the medical profession, whom I subsequently questioned about this have all said that there was no medical reason why this drug could not have been give as soon as I had arrived and been examined the night before.

I was taken up to a ward and after another couple of doctors had examined me I was told that I would be having a cat scan that morning and that there would be some more tests to be made, the results of which would be available the following day. I was assured that the pain could be easily controlled and not to worry. I felt relieved that there seemed to be no urgency about these things.

It was about ten thirty the following morning when one of the doctors who had examined me the previous day arrived with a few other white coats. He asked if I minded if a couple of them examined me and I said fine. From their youth, I presumed that they were student doctors, so in a way, I was their guinea pig. 'Very appropriate,' I remember thinking! Afterwards, they all moved away, went into a huddle and were no doubt comparing notes. The doctor came and sat down on the bed and it was clear that he was about to deliver the verdict.

I am pleased that he didn't beat about the bush. "What you have got is a growth in the left kidney which could be cancerous. It means that we have to take out the whole kidney," he begun, and then went on to explain in more depth. I am sure that I heard the first bit of his explanation but I cannot remember anything about it for my mind had gone into shock and then into defensive mode.

I say defensive but it was more a straw clutching stage for the first thought that came into my mind was this.

"Oh well, at least I am not going to suffering all the diseases of old age for this is it, I am gong to die!" It was a straw of sorts, I guess, but that word cancer in connection with myself had to be coped with somehow!

The doctor went on to explain that he was pretty certain that the growth had been caught early enough and that by removing the kidney the problem would be solved. He assured me that if he was right that I could continue to live normal life on the remaining kidney, which had been checked and found to be fine. He added that this kind of cancer was quite common in men of my age, and that in most cases like mine where the onset of symptoms had been rapid instead of a gradual deterioration of general health the prognosis was very good indeed. He told me that the operation was scheduled for two days time and then asked me if there were any questions that I wanted to ask him. I told him that I thought he had covered everything pretty thoroughly and I put myself in his hands.

My next worry was to work out how to tell my mother that I had cancer. After what she had gone through, nursing my sister to her death, I was very concerned about how she would cope with this news. I spoke to Vedra on the phone and explained the situation. She said that she had already had a couple of chats with my brother and was sure that he would be able to explain things to my mother tactfully now that there was some definite news about my problem.

The following day a registered letter arrived with fifty pounds in it. I had been in no condition to think straight on the Sunday night and I hadn't picked up my wallet. . I had mentioned this to Vedra and she had wasted no time in getting some money down to me. There was note in the letter informing me that the piggy evacuation from my flat was set in hand and that all of them would be safely up at the Trust by the end of the day. I was 'commanded' not to worry and just concentrate on getting well soon.

This was just one more example of piggy people proving how nice they are for so many of them seemed to have pitched in and lent a hand. The actual ferrying of the wee ones up to the Trust was done by a lady from Hampshire in her camper van. Other's came into my flat, cleaned out all the pens and made the place ready for the time when myself and my animals would be returning home.

During the two days before I went down for the operation I had received many cards and letters wishing me well, mainly from the guinea pig fraternity. The general gist of the sentiments were, 'you and Vedra saved the lives of our animals and we need you to carry on your work!' With that kind of support, the lopsided grin on my face as they wheeled me down to the operating theatre was not all down to the pre-med drug. I just felt that there were a lot of people out there rooting for me, and it was a good feeling.

I was given an epidural anaesthetic so for the first couple of days after the operation I was not really with it. Later, my mother told me that when my brother and had brought her up to visit me I was a bit slurry in speech and sounded as though I had had one too many. I certainly felt no pain but was well aware of what was going, as the nursing staff busied themselves about me but in a kind of detached manner.

I presume that the pain-killing drug is gradually reduced as the patient recovers from the operation and that the time it takes between patients must vary. In my case, I think that the first time I began to take a real interest in what was going on about me was on the third day. I can certainly pin point the moment!

A rather attractive Irish nurse by the name of Jenny, ample bosomed and like many of her kind an absolute sweetheart, was leaning over me adjusting my pillows and asking how I was feeling. I told her fine, and immediately

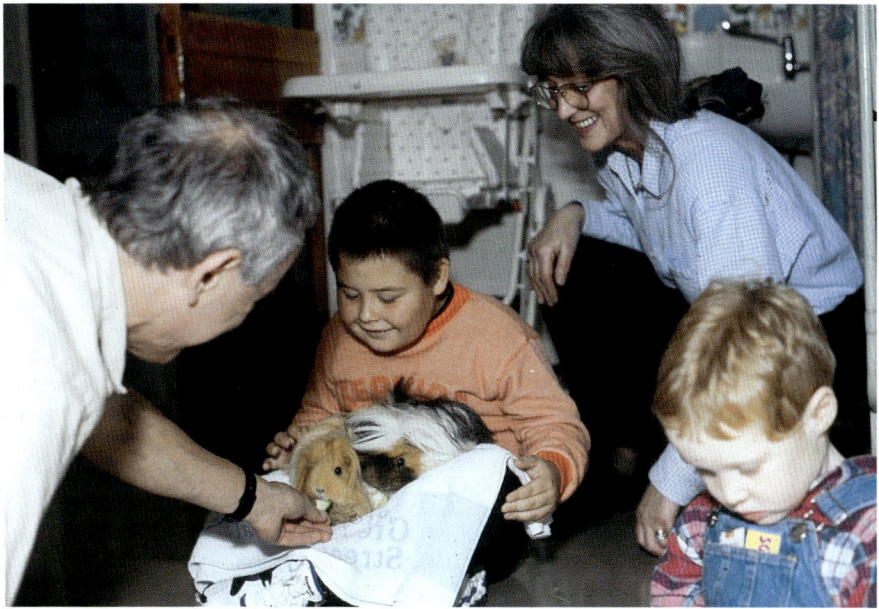

Visiting children in Great Ormond Street Hospital

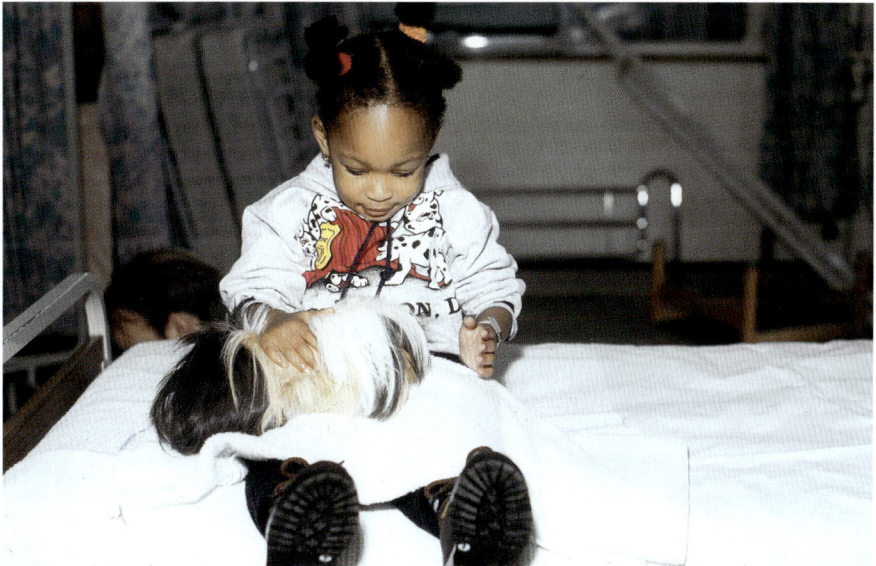

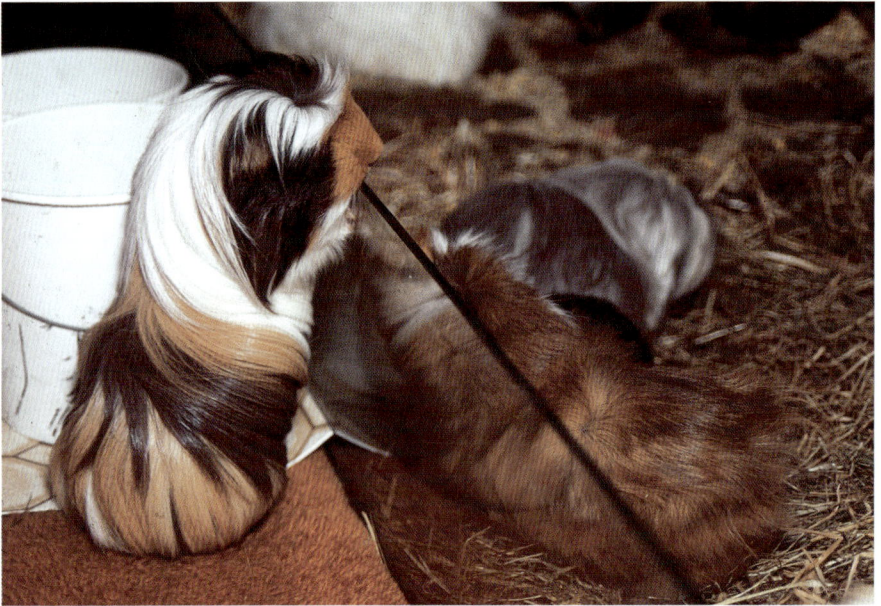

Chipper

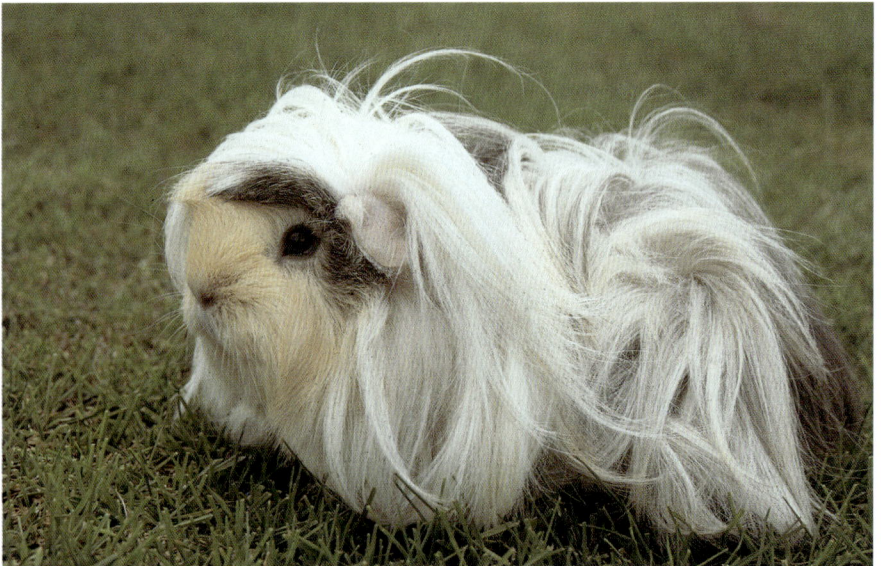

Katie

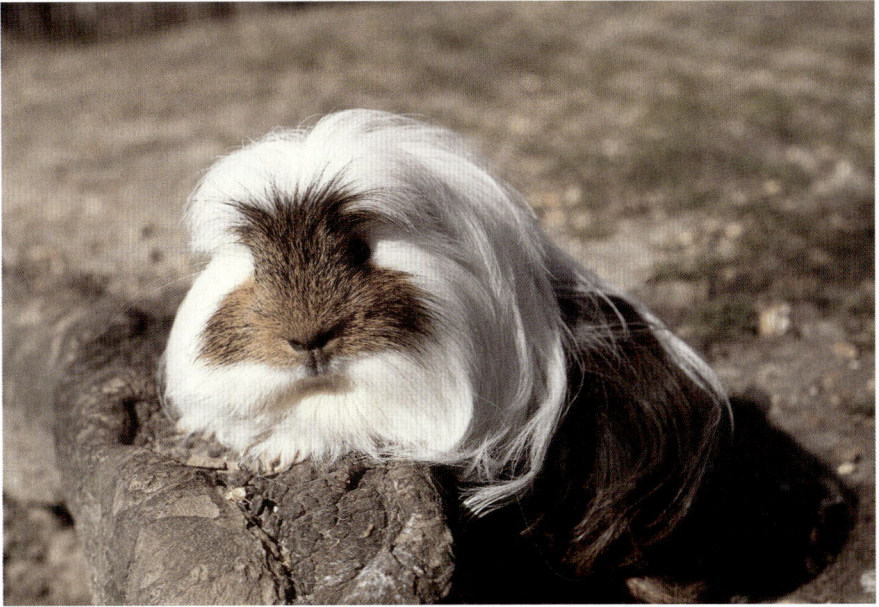

Doddy

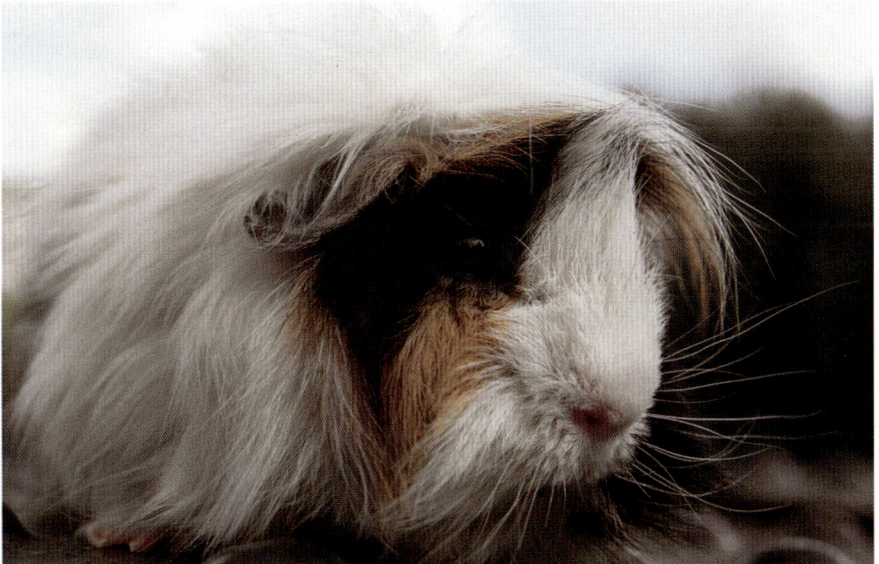

Free Range Fred

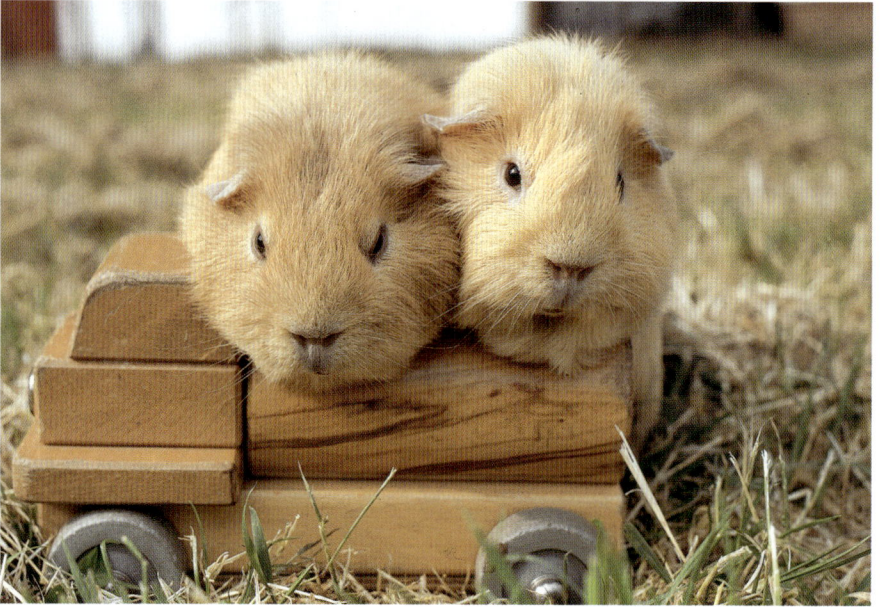

Simon & Garfunkel

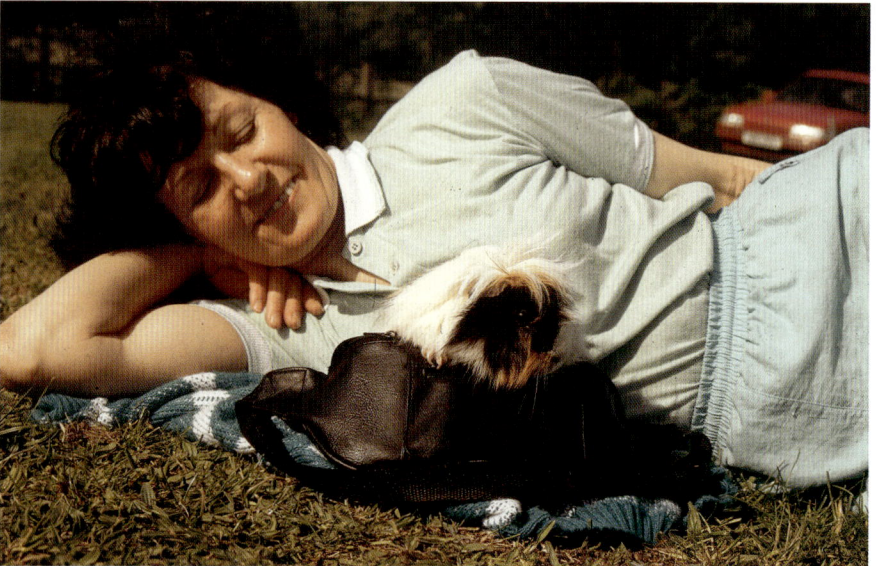

Vedra & Free Range Fred

averted my gaze, and in that split second I remember thinking to myself 'You are definitely getting better, my son!' Why? I had looked away because I was embarrassed that Jenny would catch me looking down her delicious cleavage!

Up until that moment, all the nurses could have been dancing around in attendance upon me in the nude or dressed up in the most alluring lingerie and would not have taken the slightest bit of interest! From that moment on my improvement was rapid. I think that the first time I was allowed to get up and have a proper soak in a bath was one of the most enjoyable moments of my life.

I was back home within three weeks and much to my delight I discovered that Vedra had given thought to how I would feel returning to an empty home. I had phoned to let my friend know when I would be home. As soon as I shut the front door I heard some very familiar squeaking and upon entering the living room I saw Dandy, my magnificent tri-coloured boar. He was in one of my plastic bottomed cages, standing with his forepaws gripping the wire mesh of the cage. It had been Vedra's idea my friend had told me when we spoke later that night on the phone. She had asked him to hang onto Dandy while the rest of the stock went up to the Trust so that I would have at least one guinea pig to greet me when I came home. My friend had brought him round a couple of hours before I was due.

I lifted Dandy out of the cage, snuggled him into the crook of my neck and wept like a child. Some of my tears were of pure gratitude and relief that I was still around in this living, breathing world after all. However, in the main, they were in gratitude to all the wonderful people who had been there when I needed them, and for these wonderful creatures that had made my life so much more worth living.

The icing on the cake came a couple of days later when two ladies arrived in a camper van loaded with the rest of my beasties, which they had taken up to the Trust when I fell ill. It simply didn't get any better than that, and the sight of those familiar faces settling into their pens again and checking everything out made me feel the luckiest man alive.

Fred, whom for his time up at the Trust had to undergo the indignity of living in a pen, went on a very extensive tour of inspection. He plaid particular attention to his favourite nooks and crannies, before checking out the sow pen and having what looked like a head count! For the next couple of days he spent most of his time in one of his favourite spots, a corner by the top of my futon, returning to his quarters in the kitchen only when he wanted something to eat. I have a feeling that his quarters reminded him too much of his confinement to a pen up at the Trust and he preferred the wide open spaces of my living room for a while.

Celia, my journalist friend, phoned to ask how I was, wished me well and suggested that I write to Doctor Axelrod, the head of the American publishers, TFH again. This was the world's leading publisher of books that dealt exclusively with all forms of air, land and sea life and specializing in those that were kept as pets.

I had sent Doctor Axelrod something that I had written about my life with guinea pigs about a year earlier, and much to my surprise I received a very charming, personal letter back from him. He told me how much he enjoyed my style of writing but unfortunately the books that his company published were exclusively, photographically illustrated text books. As it happened, at the time that I had first written to him I had just taken up photography and during the intervening year I had devoted a lot of time to learning as much as I could about it.

I don't know if this is a personal trait but whenever I take up a new interest, which I know will not be a passing fad, I always buy the best equipment available. I just feel that if I buy the best there is then there is no cop out. I cannot blame my tools if my work it not up to scratch. It is also a good incentive to work hard at improving my skills for having spent a lot of money I want a decent return on my investment. I have not yet worked out if this phenomenon is because I am mean or lack the confidence to finish anything I start!

I duly wrote to Doctor Axelrod and got a reply back within a week. I was asked if I would be interested in writing a book and photographically illustrating it about the care of guinea pig for a new series that his company was planning to produce.

Would I be interested! What! Interested in writing for such a prestigious publisher as TFH! He might have well have asked if I was interested in hitting the jackpot of my most vital ambition.

In retrospect, I am amazed at my confidence in my ability to take on such a task. OK, so I was certain that I could put the words together but I had only got into the photographic side of things for a year and I still regarded myself as a novice when it came to the veterinary care of guinea pigs. The advantages I had of course, were the appalling lack of knowledge by the veterinary profession of these animal's needs, being tutored by Vedra, and the kind of hands-on experience I had had of working on just this species up at the Trust. To add to this was the experience I had gained by holding surgeries at my mother's home in Luton, Bedfordshire.

I had started these Saturday morning surgeries about four months before my kidney problem. Almost all of the animals I saw belonged to owners who were appalled at the standard of care they were receiving from local vets. There were some rumblings of discontent from one of these vets when he got wind of my activities but no attempt was made to stop my work. However, it was about this time that I began to become aware that there were some absolutely brilliant vets around. Teresa and Colin had a couple and I was soon to learn of a few more.

I think that it took me about three months to put the text together of my first book, and about a month for the photographic slides. Luckily, I had been building up quite a library of slides, many of which I hoped could be used as evidence of the kind of veterinary incompetence we were dealing with. On this latter point, I can only say silly me! I thought that it would only be a matter of sending this kind of evidence to a consumer organization or a member of Parliament, or even and animal welfare organization and the R.C.V.S. would come running out of it's bunker with it's hands above it's head. After ten years of an exercise, which has been like trying to punch candy floss, I am a much wiser man now and I long ago gave up writing to politicians or any other bodies that are supposed to be responsible for animal welfare in this country. For all the talk about ethical standards, strict regulations and statutory complaints procedures, the chances the legitimate concerns of the general public being listened to yet alone acted upon are very, very slim indeed. The only thing that puzzles me is that the general public still seems to have faith in what profession people say in the light of the increasing evidence of the most gross blundering.

When the book was completed I carefully parceled it up, insured it, and sent it off to the headquarters of TFH in New Jersey U.S.A.. I was on tenterhooks until I got confirmation that it had been safely received. Of course, I had taken the precaution of making a copy of the text but I had not copies of the slides.

When the post arrived some three weeks later, anyone passing my door would have heard a great whoop of joy. There was a letter from TFH informing me that they were delighted with the typescript and slides and the made me an offer. A week later a contract arrived, which I duly signed and sent back. There was a definite spring in my step as I walked over to the post office. Goodness gracious, it looked like I was going to be a published author!

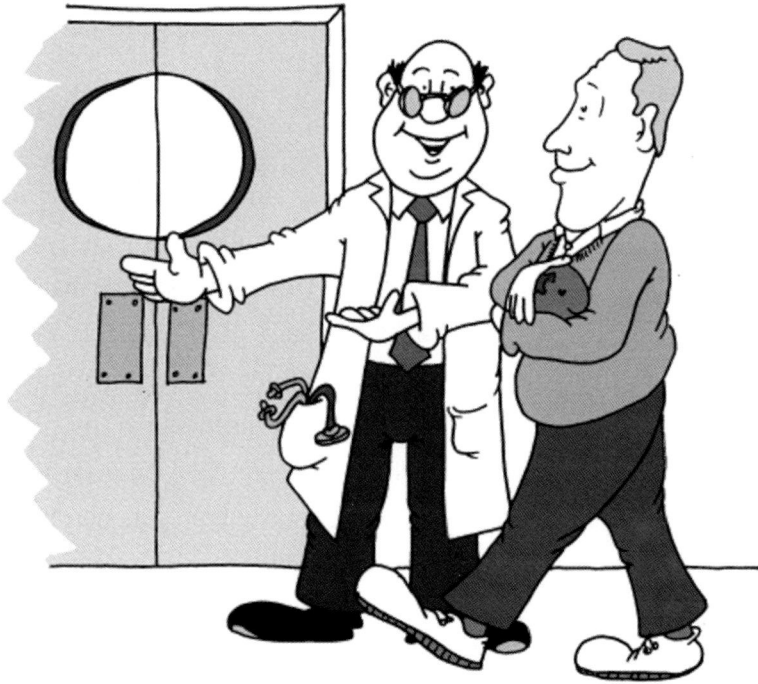

Chapter nine.

The child first, and always the child.

I like to think that the motto for G.O.S.H. is also applicable for PG's GPs, only the word guinea pig substituted for child. The more I work with the children the more I feel that what I do and what the staff of the hospital do are the same. G.O.S.H. is devoted to the care of small children while all my efforts are directed to the care of small animals. However, we both have a holistic approach to our work, hugs, t.l.c. being considered as vital a part of the treatment as all the surgical and medical expertise that we use to cure our patients.

Let me make it clear that before I started visiting the hospital I was not into children in a big way. They didn't like jazz, couldn't understand Shakespeare and played lots of noisy games. With such criteria set as a standard by myself what chance did the poor little mites stand to gain any kind of place in my popularity poll!

The one big advantage that I did have was my inability to do the coochy coo bit so right from the start I treated them as minipeople. "hi Sweetheart, or mate,' as the case maybe, was and still is my way of introducing myself to children. I had no problem with getting on down and playing with the ones that were mobile in the playrooms or simply sitting on the ward floor. I noticed that many of the staff were just as uninhibited as I was, including the male staff.

I think I should point out here that I have deep problems with modern macho man and really enjoy getting right up his testosterone stuffed nose. Many a time when I am lying on my back on the grass in the park, with a guinea pig high up on my chest with whom I am enjoying a good old nasal gaze, I have noticed a smirk of contempt, usually from younger men as they pass by. I always smile and say to myself, " you can't do this, can you, sonny. Your macho image is far more important to you than having fun. Sad!"

Macho man for me is the surgeon walking down one of the corridors from one of the operating theaters after having restored a child's hearing, sight, or perhaps carrying out a life saving operation.

All the things that my fellow men seem to enjoy proving them selves at, such as sport, trekking to the north pole or sailing across the Atlantic in a bathtub, leave me scratching my head and looking down my Y fronts to check out if I am indeed of the male sex, for I have never had the slightest desire to try any of them.

Though at first we had restricted the visiting to the play centre, we soon expanded to the wards by popular demand, and our confidence that there was nothing nasty that a guinea pig could pass onto a child.

A routine was set which has not altered down the years. On Monday evening I give the visiting guinea pigs a thorough veterinary inspection, playing particular attention to their coats. Ringworm, nothing to do with worms I hasten to add but a fungal skin condition, is about the only thing that a child could pick up from a guinea pig. For the child this would be a very minor thing and in no way threatening to it's over all health. However, any guinea pigs with the slightest sign of a skin problem, or ones that have had one in the past couple of weeks, will be automatically counted out.

Right from the early days when I had Fred, my first free ranger, the free ranger always comes along with me. Fred kind of set a precedent and all the subsequent free rangers that I have taken with me have proved to become favourites.

I get a great kick whenever one of my guinea pigs is asked for by name and don't mind in the least when I am scolded by a small child for not bringing up their particular favourite. I have to add, that on more than one occasion that I have also got it in the neck from quite a few of the nurses when their favourites are absent when they happen to be on duty!

Before we do our rounds in each ward I will check out with the head nurse to see if there are any neutropenic patients. These are patients who's resistance to infections have been impaired by their illness or as a result of surgery. These I will cross off my visiting list to avoid the lightest risk of them picking up anything from myself or my guinea pigs.

Most of the wards contain single units for individual patients on either side of a corridor that leads down to a more open plan area, which usually has three or four beds in it.

Very early on I discovered what the attitude was of most of the consultants was towards the wee beasties visiting their patients, when I was about to go into one of the small units and met one of them and his team coming out. He was a very large man, with a booming voice. As soon as he caught sight of me and my long box full of piggies he turned back to the open door of the unit and called into his patient. "Ah, now the proper doctor is coming in," then turning back to me and my box, motioned his team to stand to one side, bowed and motioned me in with an elaborate flourish of his hand.

It was also very early on that I witnessed an instance of the holistic approach to a patient by a consultant. We had been visiting a little Egyptian girl named Amira for about three weeks. She had some kind of spinal or neck injury, which meant that she had to wear a neck and head support that looked like a steel cage over her head and shoulders. She also had a tracheostomy in her neck to enable her to breath.

As soon as the consultant and his team entered the unit I reached for the piggy that Amira was nursing on her lap and made to leave, promising that I would come back later.

"Oh don't worry about us, it's only a chat we're after," said the consultant with a grin.

Amira's mother was there but I noticed that he didn't chat over Amira but went out of his way to include her in the conversation as much as possible. Just as he was about to leave, Amira said something to her mother. Though both mother and daughter spoke very good English indeed it was sometimes difficult for me to understand Amira because her speech was obviously not made easier by the tube in her windpipe. Her mother had no such problem and she turned to the consultant and said, "You know what she's asking for, of course!"

At this, the consultant, moved close to the side of the bed, took Amira,'s hand in his and made her a solemn vow.

"Amira, I promise you that when we unhook you from that lot," he said, pointing to the tubes flowing in and out of the hi tech equipment and into her, "You shall have your Coca-cola!"

Goodness knows how many patients he had but I was willing to bet that he had taken the trouble to find out as many of the fads and fancies of each and every one of them as he could.

Once, when I walked into Amira's unit, I was greeted by a Pixie, for that is what she looked like from the face painting that had been done on her. The nurse, who had her back towards me, turned when she heard my voice and I saw that she too had been face painted only she was a gorgeous marmalade pussy cat! These nurses are not only highly trained in the cutting edge of pedi-atric nursing skills they are also pretty hot in the other important skills of mak-ing the children feel that they too can 'boogie on down' and join their patients in their fun. However, as the nurses are kept very busy doing the nitty-gritty working of nursing their charges each ward has a play therapist who take on the task of full time play with the children. They also carry out vital liaison work with the patients and staff.

When I fist visited the P.I.C.U., Pediatric Intensive Care Unit, it was like walking onto the set of the film 2001 for there was gleaming white hi tech equipment all over the place. There were TV monitors a plenty, recording goodness knows what from the tiny patients. It all came out as incomprehensible, to me at least, squiggles, dots lines and numbers. The amount of equipment around each bed was awesome, as were the tubes and wires that came from it and were attached the frail looking patients.

It was obviously very labour intensive for there seemed to be double the number of staff as I had seen on the normal wards, checking and rechecking the various monitors. However, despite the high concentration of nurses and equipment the parents had not been excluded for by at the foot of each bed where easy chairs, many of which were occupied by mother or father or both.

I noticed that one of these parents was assisting one of the nurses and I later learned that they were encouraged to get involved with the nursing of their children whenever it was possible. In many cases this wasn't just a kind of therapeutic thing, which made the parents feel that they were involved. Certain procedures would have to be continued when the children were allowed home so it was important that the parents were taught them. As this is exactly what I do with the owners of sick guinea pig that are brought to me I could appreciate the value of this holistic approach.

Having had so much experience of the condescension and arrogance of so many veterinary surgeons toward the owners of animals because of their presumption that only they have knowledge or skills and that owners are simpletons, I was even more impressed by the attitude of the staff of G.O.S.H. towards parents. They obviously shared Vedra's notion when she urged her students to never under estimate the skills and willingness of owners to understand the problems their animals had and their abilities to nurse them well. This is an example of an holistic approach where everyone chips in.

Just before my first book was published in this country in 1993 we did our first T.V. stint at the hospital. This was very nice timing from my publisher's point of view but the icing on the cake was that it was good publicity for the hospital and the whole business of animal visits to hospitals in general.

The proof copy of my book, 'The Proper care of guinea pigs,' arrived on a Saturday morning when I was up at my mother's holding a surgery. I arrived back home to find a note from my postman whom I knew very well and had told about the book. He said that rather than send it back to the sorting office he had taken it across to the sub post office across the road and given it to the couple of ran it. He knew I they were friends of mine and that I would be able to pick it up as soon as they opened on the following Monday morning. The frustration of that wait till Monday morning is something I shall never forget.

There is nothing like the thrill of seeing your name on the cover of a book for the very first time and I think that I must have been walking two feet above the ground when I got back to my flat. When I opened up the parcel and scanned through the book I was delighted and surprised to see how little my text had been edited. The high quality glossy paper that the   book was laid out on really did justice to the photographs and I got a great kick out seeing so many of my guinea pig friends, past and present.

I few weeks later I got my author's free copies. The first person I sent a copy to was Jilly Cooper the author and journalist. I had recently lost her namesake, an adorable grey and blond sheltie sow, at the age of six years. I had acquired her from a local pet shop at a time when I had been reading Jilly's very amusing book about her adventures when she had been living near Barnes common in the south west of London.

The very morning that my Jilly came into my life there had been an article in a national newspaper by Jilly, carrying a photograph of her in which it could clearly be seen that her blond hair had some greying. The hair, both in style and colour matched my, as yet, unnamed sheltie. There was also a jaunty air about her, a boldness. and she looked as though she was going to be a lot of fun. Her name just had to be Jilly, after the lady who's work had made me roar with laughter so many times, particularly when it concerned her desperate struggle to control one of the many much loved but wayward dogs that enhanced her life.

When I was reading the book about the Barns common years I got through quite a few tissues, soaking up the tears of laughter that were rolling down my cheeks. In that particular book of hers, I got that feeling of 'I know just where you are coming from, lady!' as I read her reflections of life's funny ways so skillfully put into words.

I took Jilly round to a friend of mine and told her how she had got her name. She thought it was very appropriate and urged me to write to Jilly, send her a photograph of her namesake and explain why she had been so named. It took a few weeks before I got round to it but in the end I did just that.

A week later I received a very charming letter from Jilly informing me that she had had a Chrysanthemum and a racing care named after her but nothing quite as lovely as my Jilly. Throughout Jilly's life, her namesake kept up a correspondence with her!

Jilly wrote back, thanking me for the copy of the book and said that it was a wonderful memorial to her namesake for she had been featured in quite a few photographs in the book. Subsequently, the sending of a copy of my latest book to this lovely lady has become a bit of a tradition.

Later, in 1993, I was to meet another very well known personality, her owner and his wife, Sue, who have become very dear friends of mine. Her name was none other than Olga De Polga, who's adventures her creator, Michael Bond writes about. Michael is probably more well known for his other creation, the magnificent Paddington bear, and more recently, Monsieur Pamplemoose.

I had been working up at the Trust when Vedra took a call from Michael who was not at all happy about the diagnosis and treatment that his current Olga had received from his vet. I had been busy with a patient and it's owner when Vedra had passed the message on that I would be having a patient into see me when I got home the following day. I think I picked up the fact that it was a V.I.P., Very Important Piggy, but I didn't pay too much attention to just who it was or to whom it belonged.

Early the following evening a chap arrived with a box out of which he took a magnificent looking tri-coloured Abysinnian guinea pig and told me that her name was Olga. He told me that she had been off colour for a while and that his vets seemed to be floundering, trying all manner of drugs on her but getting no positive results. It was a very familiar story and I set too giving Olga a thorough examination. While I was working, Michael told me that though he knew of me through something he had read in a newspaper, it was only recently that he had been told by a friend of the C.C.T.

Machael was amazed at the thoroughness of the examination that I subjected Olga to. He shouldn't have been for I was doing no more than the basics. However, they were the basics according to the gospel of Vedra Standley-Spatcher. Needless to say they are far more thorough than could be expected from the average member of the R.C.V.S. When compared to the kind of examination that we have come to expect from the average vet of a guinea pig, there is a brief look while ours is a strip down body search! In essence, the kind of examination that Vedra trains her students to carry out can be summed up in a very succinct couple of sentences she came out with when she was talking to a student whom she thought had only done half a job.

"If a patient comes in with a sniffy nose and a bit of a chesty wheeze that looks as though it's not much more than a bit of a cold you still do the business. You examine the whole of the animal, and this includes looking up it's backside if necessary!" Vedra is never a lady for half measures.

I told Michael what I thought the problem was and to throw away everything that the vet had prescribed, all of which were prescription medicines that were the wrong ones for the symptoms I was seeing and I put her on a couple of over the counter medicines. These medicines of course, were far less expensive than those prescribed but then they usually are. They were also less likely to upset the delicate gut flora of a guinea pig, a vital factor in this particular case than those prescribed by Olga's vet. I told Michael to monitor Olga closely and bring her back to me within a couple of days if she hadn't improved.

I asked Michael if he had seen my book about guinea pig care and when he said he hadn't I showed him a copy. He seemed very impressed and thought that there was a great need for such a detailed book. He then mentioned that he would stick to books about his Olga and leave the veterinary books to experts like myself.

Somewhere at the back of my mind Vedra's voice echoed and the words De Polga rang out very clearly.

"Hang on," I said, hesitantly. "Bond! Are you Michael Bond?" I asked.

"The same," replied Michael, with a grin.

"Oh my God. So this must be THE Olga," I cried, as the realization struck me that I was responsible for the health of such a renowned little lady.

"You do realize, of course, that if I get this wrong and anything happens to Olga here that Vedra will give me a loaded revolver and tell me to go out and do the decent thing!" I pointed out, grimly.

Michael grinned and said that if the examination was anything to go by there could not have been much that I had missed.

A few days later I got a call from Sue telling me that Olga was back on top form, eating like a horse, and that her self assertive temperament was back into top gear and that she and Michael could not thank me enough.

I breathed a big sigh of relief and the net result of it all was that I took on her veterinary care and that of her successor five years later, after she died at the ripe old age of seven and a half years. Both have also boarded with me whenever the Bonds go away.

Both Michael and myself were guilty of a criminal offence when he brought Olga to me for treatment. He was breaking the law for taking an animal to someone whom he knew was not a qualified vet, and I was doing the same thing in treating it. We merrily continue to break the laws of this land for I still treat the Olgas in our lives. Our problem is that we put the health of and welfare of the animals that we are both responsible for above the proven lack of responsibility of the veterinary profession of this country to adhere to the very law that that it accuses us of breaking. In short, no matter how many fancy letters they may have after their names we do not regard the vast majority of them as being properly qualified to treat Olga or any other guinea pig. Until they do get their act together we shall continue to protect Olga against those whom we regard as a danger to her health and welfare. End of story!

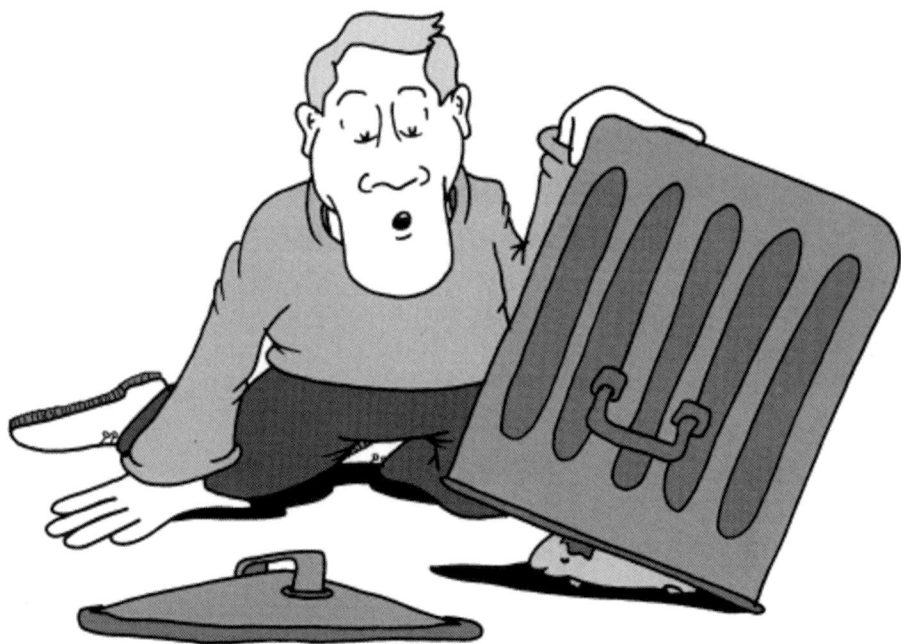

Chapter ten.

New ways and back to school.

For the life of me I cannot remember who first approached me about taking piggies to local schools and children's libraries but I do know that it was very early on in my guinea pig career.

The first thing I was to learn was that I was truly back in school myself! The first two that I visited I think I went in with the idea that I was just going to get up, wave a couple of guinea pigs about and walk out unharmed. Mistake! I quickly learned that I had to play a class of children like a theatre audience, say, or in some cases like a hostile crowd at Speaker's corner! You have to be prepared to give as good as you get when they decide that a wee bit of audience participation will liven things up a bit for if you don't hit back they will eat you alive!

In those early day I needed a teacher to hand all the time to keep order for I didn't have a clue. It's all about pacing and how to go along with the flow when it's going in the direction that you want it to go. If you don't grab their interest right from the start or quickly change tack when you think that you are losing them then it can begin with fidgeting and end with a kind of whip and chair job with your back to the wall!

I gradually learned that the best way to settle children down was to grab their interest in anecdotes about my animals before I got some serious facts into their heads. They particularly enjoyed ones where a human being, especially if it was an adult one, was made the butt of a guinea pig's joke. Having lived with guinea pigs for so long there was certainly no need of invention on this score for more often than not in the guinea pig-human battle of wills it is the human that ends up with egg all over it's silly face!

It was better to hold back before opening up the traveling box to reveal the 'goodies.' If I was premature on this score they were not likely to want to switch back to the 'boring old adult waffling on' mode. When I did take out my first guinea pig I had to ensure that it was relevant to a point was leading up to or one that I had just made. If I didn't get this right I would soon be distracted and lose my thread, being asked all manner of questions about guinea pig life and care and some that had absolutely nothing to do with guinea pigs. There is nothing like floundering about under the gaze of a sea of mocking children's faces when at the time you thought you were being ever so clever and informative and in full control. It quickly teaches you that you have completely lost the plot and sometimes that you never had one right from the start!

When it comes to question time, after you have primed them properly, the rewards can be tremendous, even when sometimes you cannot answer a particular question. On more than one occasion when I have found that I have been stumped I had to say to myself, 'now why didn't I ask that question years ago?' Children have a different perspective on things and I have learned quite a lot by having to seek out answers to some of the questions that they have put to me that I could not answer at the time.

In any group of children you will always get one! The one who thinks that it's a really good career move to trip up the adult who has taken it upon himself to lecture them. Nine times out of ten the career that they are trying to enhance is the one that defines their place in the pecking order of the pack! I am pleased to say that I have become quite skilled at detecting them very early on in the proceedings. I mentally mark their card and am usually ready to counter their attempts to phase me!

The most common first thrust, usually from a boy in an older class group is "How do you tell the difference between a girl and a boy guinea pig?"

I smile sweetly and ask, "How old are you, sonny?"

The question is usually unexpected and before he gets chance to answer it I go in for the coup-de-grace by very rapidly adding, "I would have thought that a lad of your age would know the difference between girls and boys by now." Drop a few positions in the pecking order sonny as the rest of the class laugh at him!

The girl 'ones' are usually a bit more subtle but the theme is usually the same and with the main aim of embarrassing me

"Do girl guinea pigs have periods?" an innocent looking girl once asked, all sweetness, one day.

You use a different tack on these kind of questions.

"Not quite like human beings but they do have something called an estrus cycle, which runs for about half the monthly term for the female of the human species."

This, delivered po-faced, and in a dull boring manner that sounds as though it could go on far too long, is not half as juicy as expected. This kind of reply usually puts the questioner off their stroke and the ball is back in my court!

Though I like to think that I have developed my lecturing technique off to a fine art I still get caught out now and again, which is very good for me for it stops me getting too complacent and consequently, stale. The best compliment upon my technique was from a police sergeant who had been sitting at the back of the hall when I had been talking to a complete assembly of children one   morning. He came up to me afterwards and said, with a very pained expression on his face.

"Do me a favour. Try and avoid coming and doing your bit before I have to do mine in future. In fifteen minutes time I have to grab their attention and hold it on the 'exciting' topic of road safety .How can I follow and act like yours?" I told him to get some good props, such a couple of guinea pigs, perhaps!

The talks I give in libraries were much easier for they usually followed a story telling session by one of the library staff so my audience was well settled by the time I got them. In both the schools and the libraries we allowed the children to handle the guinea pigs by dividing them into small groups, sitting them down in circles and putting a piggy in the middle. I always took some tit-bits of green food with me so that the children could feed their particular piggy. This way, the children were easy to monitor and I'm pleased to say that in all the time that I have been doing this work we have never had any accidents with a guinea pig.

In 1993 a bill was being discussed in Parliament, which though claiming to have the aim of improving the safety of medicines for animals was nothing but a measure to tighten up, even more, the monopoly of the R.C.V.S. over the treatment of animals.

It was to be called the veterinary medicines act and was to ban the use of any drug that had not been licensed for use upon animals, even if an identical drug was proved to be safe and effective for use upon humans. One or two vets who still retained some kind of ethical standards had the guts to stand up and be counted and protest against the proposed legislation. They pointed out, and in the event they have proven to be correct, that this measure would put up the already high cost of veterinary medicines even more. However, as the legislation had been proposed by the veterinary profession's top so called experts in the first place the majority of vets supported it and it became law in 1994. The same old sad story of keeping a united front, obviously.

I believe that this is yet one more law that has added to the increasing infringement of our civil liberties in that it interferes with a citizen's right to diagnose and treat their own animals. Incidentally, at the time of writing, the next move against our freedoms is brewing away in Parliament by a paper put forward by that anachronism, 'The house of fossils,' proposing legislation to bring all alternative medicines under similar laws. Great news for the bank balances of the drug companies and professions engaged in conventional medical and veterinary care but one more nail in the coffin of our rights to make our own decisions about the way we lead our lives. Nanny State is a busy old Bitch these days!

I recently wrote to one of the figures concerned with his kind of nannying, asking him if he thought it was possible to set up a focus group to look into the feasibility of getting some research done into the quality of toilet paper. We could maybe get a research grant made to one of our 'great centres of learning' to do a study into, a much neglected part of the life of the nation. Yes, it will be only a matter of time before some cretin in some ministry or another will come to the conclusion that none of us know how to wipe our own backsides without professional advice or special aids! I never did get a reply; perhaps they are at it, even now, setting up committees and taking advice from the white coats!

The argument put forward to justify this kind of outrageous legislation is that all medicines have to be scientifically tested to prove that they are safe and effective. Fine, but even back in the early nineties when this nonsense began, myself and many other people were beginning to have serious concerns about the close ties between the professions the legislators and the drug companies. The Thalidomide debate and the failure of so many other drugs that had been through all the 'thorough' scientific testing put serious doubts into our minds about the wisdom and trustworthiness of politicians and their advisers. The subsequent BSE disaster and increased diseases in cattle has certainly not increased our confidence in the reliability of government experts to get things anywhere near right.

Because of the monopoly that vets had on most animal medicines before the 1994 law came into force I had already begun researching into alternative and over the counter medicines for animals. I already knew that many, though not all, alternative drugs that were formulated for use upon humans were also safe and effective for use upon animals. However, the deeper I got into it the wider was the choice, far wider than I thought it would be.

Now, early in 2002, how tempting it is to say, 'I told you so' when I heard the recent news that as a result of many pet owners complaining about the high cost of veterinary medicines that a commission of enquiry is to be set up into these prices!]

It was at about this time that I began to write the R.C.V.S. and many other authorities to air mine and the concerns of many other people about the standard of veterinary care available in this country. Foolishly, I continued to do so up until about a year ago when I decided to write this book. I guess I am a slow learner for right from the start it was made abundantly clear to me that the opinions of myself and those that I spoke for were simply not valid. That attitude was, and still is, 'Go away little man and get some letters after your name." This deplorable level of closed mindedness is symptomatic of very many professions in this country and the reason why the level of profession services in this country is far lower than in those of many other countries.

I have forgotten the number of times that I have said to an owner, "He or she is either an Australian, New Zealander, or Continental vet" when they have told me that either, A, they were honestly uncertain of what the problem was, or B, had carried out a proper examination and got very close to a correct diagnosis. The times when it has been a British vet are very rare indeed! The average British vet still believe that only he or she has the training to treat animals and never, ever admit that they do not know.

By early 1994 I had sufficient information to set about writing 'Piggy Potions,' my second book. Needless to say, I consulted Vedra at every stage when it came to the subject of conventional medicines and as in all my books she was given credit on the first page for the veterinary information contained therein.

One of the most rewarding result of my researches was the discovery of an alternative treatment for the many common skin conditions that guinea pig flesh is heir to. Despite their access to all the modern diagnostic techniques the failure of the average high street vet to differentiate between fungal and parasitic skin conditions is a disgrace and results in the suffering and death of many guinea pigs. I put this down to the very reliance on these modern techniques. In our opinion the veterinary colleges should spend a great deal more time teaching their students to rely more upon the most effective diagnostic tools of all; the nose, the eyes and a sense of touch.

Myself and anyone trained at the C.C.T., can pick up a piggy and after a brief examination, determine if it is suffering from a parasitic, fungal or hormonal problem to account for a skin problem. We do not need skin scraping and expensive laboratory tests, all of which take time, so we can begin treatment right away. Though there are safe and effective conventional treatments for these conditions, I now only use alternative treatments in the shape of an essential oil formula that I perfected and was able to publish in my Piggy Potions book. .

The vast majority of conventional practitioners in both the veterinary and medical fields get very sniffy about the use of essential oils, if the pun can be excused! They use terms, like, 'unproven' 'it's all airy fairy nonsense' and the like. I have now come to the conclusion that this is merely a manifestation of their conviction that after five years in a veterinary or medical college that only their opinions should be given credence. This line of thinking, of course, totally ignores the fact that I cannot afford to be 'airy fairy'. I am running a refuge where practical hands on work and complete confidence in the medicines that I use are the only weapons I have to ease the suffering of the animals I am responsible for. I am also not in the privileged position whereby I am protected from outside scrutiny by a powerful organization which is run by, and for, the benefit of my peers. The main regulation I have over my work is far more exacting, it is my conscience and my pride in my reputation as a healer of these adorable animals.

There is one other overwhelming controlling interest and that is my empathy with the owners who love these animals as much as I do. I have shed far too many tears over the deaths of so many of my own animals not to have a firm understanding of the kind of bond there is between these animals and their owners.

The attitude of far too many vets was expressed by a very famous T.V. vet when she was asked the question.

"Don't you feel that people who bring tiny animals to you and spend a lot of money trying to get them better rather silly?"

Even though my opinion of this woman was not good, and my expectations of her very low, even I didn't expect the succinct reply, "Well, yes!"

The fact that there was not a public outcry at this total lack of any kind of ethical standard and the callous disregard for the feelings of small animal owners was not at all surprising. It is a shining example of just how confident this woman, and many of her kind with the letters R.C.V.S. after their names, are that they can disregard their client's feelings and put down small animals as lesser creatures! Charming!

It was while I was writing Piggy Potions that the adorable Doddy came into my life. I don't think there is anything after this life, other than oblivion but if there is an after life then I am not interested in living it unless Doddy, and so many more of his kind are there waiting for me. They were my wonderful free rangers.

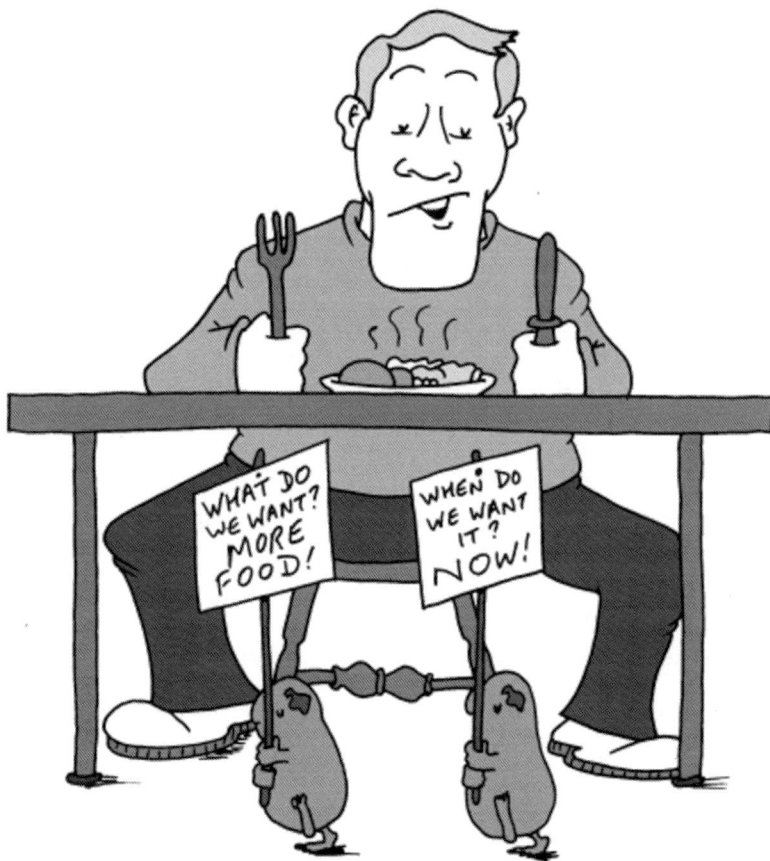

Chapter eleven.

Fred and the rest of the free rangers.

I have been in love far more times than I care to remember. I think I loved well and certainly enjoyed these affairs, despite the inevitable pain when they all came to an end. I loved that thrill when the lady who had captured my heart slipped into my mind during the working day, triggering off a silly grin of contentment on my face. The cinema of my mind would begin putting out trailers of delights to come of flashbacks of moments when the pair of us had reveled in one another. What was so wonderful about the many ladies coming and going in my life was the sheer variety of the things that I loved about them.

Though, while my current love was in my mind, we would be engaged in all manner of sexual activity, in the main it was the mundane that moved me the most. Opening my front door and seeing her standing there, smiling. Listening to her talking about her day's work or enthusing over something she was going to buy for herself. Sitting next to her in the theatre and either laughing or being moved by something in the action of the play. Sharing our views on the world, sometimes begging to differ or laying down the law about how wonderful it would be if we were ruling it! The wave over our shoulders as either she or I drove from one another's homes. The good-byes that anticipated the Hello hugs that our next date would always begin with. These were the wonderful installments of a love affair that I always savoured and that stuck in my memory making me jump back onto the merry-go-round not too long after things had gone pear shaped the last time!

Needless to say, I could not share many of these pleasures with the free ranger loves of my life but some I could and I loved them all with the same intensity. However, like the women in my life the free rangers were very individualistic and their differing traits defined them in the same way as those of the ladies that I had loved and lost.

* * * * * * * *

The first free ranger was the famous Fred, who's acquisition I have already described earlier. I get many nice comments from my American readers about my books but the most pleasing remark I ever heard was one about Fred who's photo was featured so much in Proper care of guinea pigs. I was told that many Americans who have free rangers took to calling them Freds, which gave me a great buzz for the lad deserved to be remembered.

Fred and myself were really 'guinea pigs' for one another in learning to live together and there were some very close calls in the early days. Being such a friendly cove he tended to get under my feet and was kicked a few times, not seriously but enough to evoke a very aggressive teeth rattling response. It was after he had nearly given me a hernia for the umpteenth time as

I swayed, tottered and twisted muscles in trying to redirect my momentum that anger came up with a good solution. As soon as I was firmly on two feet I yelled at him and stamped my feet. Sensibly enough, friend Fred got the hell out of there P.D.Q. My immediate reaction was to feel very guilty about losing my rag, pick him up and make a fuss of him. However, somewhere at the back of my mind my father's words about the correct way to train dogs came into my mind. "You must let them know they did wrong. They look upon you as a big dog so growl, bark or just yell as soon as they have done something wrong.

From that then on out, with Fred and with every subsequent free ranger, I made it a habit to stamp my feet, not only if the guinea tripped me but if he got too close during the first couple of weeks of free ranging. In every case, they have always cottoned on very quickly and as soon as the size nines got anywhere near them they would run for cover, usually to the nearest wall. Some took longer than others to understand that this wasn't the PP being throwing a wobbly but just being cautious and for a few days these would run and hide as soon as I entered any room they were in but they all grew out of this in the end.

Fred came with me every time I had to go up to the Trust and was allowed free range in Vedra's living room and of course, was the first free ranger to visit the hospital.

He was once nearly thrown out with the rubbish! I live on the first floor of a two story block of flats. Though on my floor there is a chute down which rubbish can be put, leading to two large six foot high bins, the plastic sack that I put the debris in from pen cleaning are too large to go in so I have to carry them down two short flights of stairs.

One day, just as I was lifting the sack to throw it over into the one of the bins I heard a rustle, a distinct sound of movement from within it. I put it on the ground, undid the top and immediately saw the brown bum of friend Fred. It was clear what had happened. These sacks were prone to fall over and lie on their sides when I was cleaning, and on this occasion Fred must have got a whiff of the 'lovely' scent of sow coming from the debris in the sack and thought he would check it out to see if there was a sow or three who would be obliging!

Bad luck, my son. There are none in there," I said, as I lifted him out with a feeling of great relief that he had made his presence known just before I was about to be unceremoniously dumped in the bin.

I had had Fred for about a year when he died and Vedra was pretty sure that it was liver damage, caused by the over medication of his former owner that caused his premature death.

There was quite a gap before Chipper, my second free ranger took over from Fred, though he was living with me for about a year in a pen with a couple of sows for I was determined to breed from him.

Chipper was one of my favourite breeds' of guinea pig, a long haired coronet. Like Fred he was a tri-colour and I had been trying to get one of his breed since I had fallen in love with Snowball, a pure white, dark eyed coronet that Vedra had owned. I am pretty certain that my love was not reciprocated. The first thing I would do after I had said hello to Vedra at the Trust each time I arrived would be to trot down the block and say hello, and have a hug with Snowball. Her reaction each and every time she heard me would be to hide under the hay and there was a distinct attitude of, 'Oh no, not him again!' about the way she looked at me as I dug her out and picked her up.

The day I went over to pick Chipper up from a friend of Vedra's who bred coronets I was as excited as a small boy on Christmas morning. I had been waiting for about six months for him and had seen him once soon after he had been born.

Needless to say he was soon introduced to my mother when I took him home with me for my Saturday surgeries and she became as smitten with him as I was. The reason I didn't put him free range at first was that I desperately wanted to breed from him. Within a couple of months, though I couldn't get another suitable Coronet, I managed to obtain two adorable sister sows, cream and white shelties, Muffet and Mandy who at five and a half months of age were old enough for breeding. All three settled down in yet another additional pen after about five months, Muffet produced three babies, all sows.

I put Chipper free range shortly after I was certain that Muffet was pregnant and he took to his freedom as though it was nothing more than his right and due. In a short while I put Mandy down with him, but she made it clear from the start that she was not at all keen on the 'wide open spaces' of my flat, so I put her back with her sister.

My mother was delighted by the way that Chipper seemed to regard her flat as his second home each time we arrived, find his favourite nooks and crannies and he quickly worked out that an eighty year old lady was a much easier push over when it came to scrounging extras that his owner!

There is a lovely spot, Sharpenhoe Clappers, high in the Chiltern hills, just north of Luton where my mother used to take my sister and I when we were children and, subsequently, her grandchildren. As soon as I was old enough to ride a bike and could be trusted out on the roads alone, I spent a great deal of my time up there and it has remained a very special place for me.

I remember quite a few visits that mother, myself and Chipper made up there during his short lifetime. There was something quite wonderful about myself, a middle aged man, sharing with his aging mother and a greatly loved pet, a spot that I had enjoyed so much when I had been a child. In the childhood visits there was usually the current pet dog running at our heels.

In these latter visits, the boy in me would come surging to the surface as we climbed the wooded hillsides of the Clappers. Mother, in her early eighties, was a lot slower then, pausing to catch her breath more than she had had to do when I was a child but still in pretty good condition for her advancing years. I felt closer to her during these times than I had ever been in my life before and my only regret was that my father could not have shared them. He had died in 1963 at the young age of sixty one. I had been a bit of a wild child and my father and I were often at odds and it was only towards the latter end of his life that I began to appreciate just how much I owed him and my mother and we were beginning to become reconciled.

I took Chipper everywhere with me, to St James and Regents Park, on all my photographic trips and even when I went over to the common for the daily ration of grass, the lad came with me. On one occasion, long after he had gone, his ghost was to cause me a great deal of embarrassment! He collected hearts the way, in my childhood, small boys collected stamps and in the two and half short years of his life he had enough to fill many albums.

He was my first, and hopefully, last guinea pig to die of a gut torsion. I noticed him looking very uncomfortable and bloated in his quarters and upon closer examination I could see that he was beginning to froth at the mouth .I phoned Vedra and she told me to get him up to the Trust as soon as possible. I left him with her and hurried back to London where I had to get back to work.

She phoned me that evening and told me that he had died during the afternoon. Though she thought she knew what had caused his death but if it wasn't what she thought then perhaps we could learn more if we had an autopsy done on him and would I give my permission. I readily agreed for apart from the fact that I have no sentimental attachment to the dead bodies of either animals or humans, the bottom line of a chance of increasing our knowledge was the number one priority and he was sent to the Newmarket Trust for the autopsy.

The pathologist who carried out the work reported back within a day that it was what Vedra had suspected, a gut torsion, one of roughly one hundred and sixty degrees and unless the animal had been dropped he could not say why this had occurred. He said that there had been no sign of the other thing that can cause this problem in ruminants, which is something stuck in the gullet that causes the animal to reach and the resulting strain resulting a twisting of the gut. He said that even in large animals such as horses that the Newmarket Trust specialized in, it wasn't an easy job to surgically correct this condition so it was virtually impossible in an animals such as a guinea pig and he would always advise that they be put down as soon as they had been diagnosed.

I was so heart broken at the unexpected death of Chipper that it was over a year before I could even bring myself to think about having another free ranger. However, when I did get one, he turned out to be the most beautiful guinea pig I have ever owned and an even more adept heart collector than his illustrious predecessor.

Of all the guinea pigs that I have loved, I think that Doddy had the most lasting impression upon me. I can still feel the tears welling in my eyes whenever one of my current guinea pigs does something in a way that Doddy did it.

Doddy arrived, along with his brother, with the most elegant guinea pig accommodation that I have ever set eye on. It was nothing less than a guinea pig Wendy house. Though the brother was quite a stunner as well, Doddy stood out as the dominant one and was by far the most pretty of the pair. He had a self assured, regal, elegant air about him that made you feel that you should be very respectful when in his presence. In any other animal these qualities would invariably be accompanied by a haughty manner and 'touch me not' tendencies. However, Doddy was a huge fan of the human species, especially when being hugged by one of them and was not in the least vane. There was a clownish quality about him with a touch of a jack the lad.

The brothers got their names from a horse feed that I sometimes feed my guinea pigs with made by the company Dodson and Horrels, shortened to Doddy and Horrors.

Doddy's hair style was particularly spectacular. He had long luxuriant locks all over, which culminated in a lion-like mane that fountained down from the crown of his head, cascading over his shoulders. In Doddy's case this mane was highlighted all the more by it's pristine whiteness against the golden agouti face and jowls and the dark gun metal grey of his back. When he walked, his hair seemed to flow in a very similar way to that of an Afgan hound.

Nowadays, sometimes when I am visiting G.O.S.H. and staff are praising a particularly gorgeous guinea pig of mine, if there is one of the staff around who knew Doddy in his day within ear shot they will usually say with very fond recall, "Ah, but you didn't know Doddy!" All who knew him felt very privileged to be around when he walked the wards.

Doddy simply didn't amble into a ward or anywhere for that matter, he always made a grand entrance. So impressive were these entrances of his that instead of taking him out of his traveling box and putting him into a child's lap, as was my normal routine, I took to putting him on the floor at the doorway and letting him sweep in, all panache and swank! Most of his female friends asked how long it took to groom all that luscious hair to get such an impressive styling. All were green with envy when I told them that I never even took a comb to him and the it was all Doddy's own work.

Much to my chagrin, though during the time that I had him I must have put a dozen sows free ranging with him, he never managed to sire a litter. There was certainly nothing wrong with his sex drive for the sight of Doddy in high rut and hot pursuit of a sow was a very familiar one during the wonderful two years that that I had him. In all cases but one the sows shared Doddy's enthusiasm and the chase was merely part of the game and not meant nor taken seriously by the Dod as a sign of her disinterest in the lad's advances. When coition did occur, and it did very frequently, the sow would splay her back legs, back onto him and make it very clear that she was very willing and able to oblige such a handsome suitor!

A female friend of mine was present once when Doddy and one of his sows were doing their stuff and on this occasion the sow in question was as mop coated as Doddy. After watching the energetic spectacle for a while she managed to splutter out, sides shaking with laughter, and tears rolling down her cheeks, "It's like watching a pair of super charged animated mops mating. Something out of the Muppets! Look at her, the brazen hussy," she added, pointing to the way that she sow was wriggling her bottom as Doddy thrust away, forepaws locked around her waist.

"Good, ain't he!" I remarked, proudly. "None of your 'wham bang and thank you Mam' with our Dod. They always go home with a smile on their faces after they've been thoroughly Doddied!"

"Well, if she isn't pregnant after that little lot you can't say that they didn't do their very best!" she added, with admiration.

Unfortunately she wasn't. I don't think there is any doubt about that fact that the fault lay with Doddy who must have been firing blanks for three sows that he definitely mated with went on to have babies with other boars.

I had only owned Doddy for about six months when he nearly met a nasty end and I would have been the author of it! One evening, I was about to go out to my local super market when, for some reason, I cast my eye about the flat to see where Doddy was. Within a few minutes and in growing panic, I came to the conclusion that he had gone AWOL. My mind immediately went back to the incident that had happened with free range Fred in the rubbish sack.

The flash back to that quickly went fast forward to that morning when I had been cleaning out the sow pens as usual. I thought I had learned the lesson from Fred's narrow escape and I either kept the refuse sack on my futton as I worked or if it was on the floor I made sure that it remained upright. However, I was aware that sometimes it did fall over and I could be lax in standing it back up again.

Grabbing a torch, I went through my front door like some mad thing, hitting the landing at a run, went down the stair three at a time and fetched up against the refuse bins like one of those cartoon characters hitting the brakes at the last second. The reason for my haste was because I had suddenly remembered all the banging and crashing that I had been hearing from a flat further along the landing. The tenant had recently died and the flat was being completely stripped out and redecorated for the next occupant.

When I had thrown the sack in the bin that morning they were almost empty. Now, to my horror, they were almost full of builder's rubbish, some of which was in the shape of shards of broken glass, plaster and sharp edged broken floor tiles. The vision of a speared, crushed and suffocated Doddy swirled in my mind, vying with frozen Doddy for it had been a bitterly cold winter's day.

With great difficulty, I managed to lower the bin down onto it's side and began, very, very gingerly to remove the building rubbish out of it. I paused every so often and listened for any sound of movement, like the member of rescue team at the site of an earthquake.

When I finally uncovered the sack, it was clear that it had burst open when it had hit the bottom of the bin. I pulled on of the torn edges and it split the whole of the sack open and some of the rolled up newspapers containing the debris from the cleaning spilled out. Out of the end of one of them I saw the very familiar face of Doddy looking up at me, blinking in the light of the torch beam.

Apart from the fact that he looked a tad disheveled with the locks of his magnificent mane hanging over his face, he didn't appear to be unduly concerned about his predicament. However, I think I detected a air of 'Well, you took your damned time about it, didn't you!" on his face.

I crawled right in, unrolled the newspaper that Doddy was in, took him into my arms and hugged him, saying his name over and over again. I am sure that if a stranger had come across us they would have called the police or perhaps the ambulance service to remove this madman to a place of safety.

I rushed the lad back up to the warmth of my flat, gave him a quick check over then settled him back into his quarters in the kitchen, while I went back downstairs to clear up the mess I had made. When I returned, Doddy was back in the living room, standing up with his forepaws hooked over the sow pen, checking them all out.

"Listen, old buddy of mine. Leave them alone they are the ones that got you into this mess, mate!" I told him.

His current sow, who I remember was a little cutie by the name of Nedine, was sitting a few feet away from him, sniffing in his direction now and again with an air of disapproval on her face!

"He'll never learn will he Nedine," I said, scooping her up and giving her a hug. "I should put him on short rations tonight!"

Doddy had been stuck in that bin for about eight hours and though there was the soiled hay for him to nibble on it was not the kind of daytime fare that he was accustomed to. For much of the rest of that evening he had his head stuck into his feeding bowl, no doubt making up for the loss of so much precious munching time! Later that evening yet one more indignity was heaped upon him in the shape of a bath. Though, unlike some of his fellow piggies he was not a "hey this damned fool is trying to drown me' merchant when being bathed he did not enjoy being soaped up, rinsed down and then towel dried. However, if it was colder than usual, with such a heavy coat as he had I felt the electric hair dryer was essential and he absolutely loved it. Needless to say he got it that night for the guilt was hanging heavily upon me. His coat always had a wonderful sheen to it after it had been blow dried and as he seemed to be making more and more appearances he was used to getting more and more of these treats.

In the Richard and Judy Good Morning programme he was publicly shamed when the whole country learned how he had cost me fifty pounds by eating my contact lenses. On Fortean TV he behaved with great decorum and grace, even though they filmed him having a bath in my kitchen sink. However, it was when he was filmed for a couple of programmes of him doing his stuff up at G.O.S.H. that he really behaved like the super star he was. I swear he knew which camera he was on and played to it like an old pro.

Doddy was also the most patient and superb photographic model that I have ever had the privilege to photograph. David Bailey himself could not have wished for a more willing and expert one. Time and time again I would set Doddy up in a pose, take my position behind the camera, put the first pressure on the shutter button, then a slit second before I pressed it he would give me just that little bit more. He would raise his head a fraction or shift his body slightly, giving me just that little bit more than I had been expecting.

The 'Doddy eye' became a talking point in the photos that I took of him and certainly enhanced my reputation as a photographer of guinea pigs. The expression "the eyes seemed to follow you around the room of gallery' when applied to the work of a portrait painter could equally apply to many of the shots I took of Doddy. However, I think it wasn't so much as down to my skills as a photographer as to Doddy's modeling expertise. He seemed to have an uncanny sense of timing, knowing just when to look directly into the lens at the split second when the shutter was released.

A friend recently gave me a video tapes of some of the things we did for

T.V. on which there was a sequence of Dod and myself at full throttle during one of our photographic sessions. It took place at the end of a long day's filming. I had settled the Dod down by the trunk of an ornamental cherry tree in the grounds beneath my flat and the producer had told the sound crew that they could pack up their equipment.

Myself and a couple of professional photographers whom I have watched photographing my guinea pigs, have had a tendency to prompt them in the same way as we would a human fashion model. This is a lot of the 'Hold it, hold it, yes!' 'A bit more, a bit more! and the like, most of which, of course, went right over the heads of the average guinea pig, the results relying much more on luck and our abilities to judge what the subject was going to be doing at the split second when we hit the shutter button. Dod, on the other hand, seemed to respond. O.k., so it would probably be in his own time but respond he would for I think he loved the attention.

Once the producer heard me doing my stuff he decided that he just had to get it on sound as well as vision and told the sound crew to set up again. In the resulting video the cameraman and the sound crew managed to capture those magic moments when Doddy and I were doing our stuff. Neither of us were in any way phased by being filmed, so absorbed were we in our own filming. At the end of the sequence I can be seen scooping up the lovely lad in my hands, holding him a few inches from my face and babbling my delight, "Doddy, my son, you are a born poseur but I don't care 'cause I love you to bits and a little more!"

I am convinced that it was the human flu virus that took my darling Doddy from me and I can pin point the time when he picked it up. There had been a particularly virulent strain doing the rounds at that time in December 1995. A family arrived with a young child who had what sounded like the early symptoms of a cold and I foolishly let her play with Doddy while I lanced an abscess in the family Guinea pig. I should have known better but I do now, banning people who have suspects colds or flu from visiting. I'll take their sick animals in at my front door but ask them to wait outside.

The following evening I was due to go up to the Trust. It was to attend a combined social and award giving event for our fist batch of rodentology students. It was late in the afternoon when I noticed that Doddy was not looking at all well and when I picked him Up I discovered that he had bad diarrhoea. I immediately phoned Vedra, describing the symptoms and their rapid onset.

"He hasn't been handled by anyone who has had this flu that's been going around, by any chance?" she asked.

I was about to say no when I remembered the little girl of the night before and told about her.

"Hm, it could well be that and we'll have to act quickly if it is."

At this time I didn't have the brilliant vet that I have now and there wasn't one that I was willing to trust to make a correct diagnosis and to prescribe the appropriate drug.

As speed was of the essence I left for the Trust right away, returning in the evening with the syringes of anti biotic. Vedra warned me that the prognosis was not good and when I got back home I could see that Doddy's condition had deteriorated. I injected him and managed to get some fluid down him, made him as comfortable as possible in a cage that had been positioned over a purpose made electric heating pad and hoped for the best.

I got up during the night to check on him but he had gone, and as rigour mortis had already set in I think he must have died shortly after I had put him back into the cage.

I made myself a cup of tea and sat in the kitchen with Doddy cradled in my lap, crying my eyes out at the prospect of Christmas without my darling Doddy. I had invested so much love into that adorable little creature and the fact that he had died at the same young age as predecessor, Chipper, had seemed to twist the knife even more. The lines that I had written about Chipper kept echoing in my mind and they were an epitaph that they now share.

Dance in my mind.

I can feel you still, snuggled into the crook of my neck,

Your body warm, through the cushion of your luxuriant locks.

I can hear you still, your whimpers of welcome, when I came
home.
Your purrs of pleasure when my fingers gently brushed your
back.

I can smell you still, meadow sweet, of the hay where you
slumbered,
Unaware of the way your sleeping contentment warmed my
heart.

I can speak of you still, for you scamper and dance in my mind,
Like you did down the days of the little life you lived with me.

Both Chipper and Doddy were tri-colours and the important lesson I learned from them was never to replace a free rangers with one that has any physical resemblance to it's predecessor. When Doddy first went free range, seeing him chuntering about in some of Chipper's favourite places and invariably making comparisons between the pair of them was painful to me and not fair to either of them. The fact that I lost them so early brought back the memories of their early days and hammered the lesson home.

Teddy Teddimous was the first Rex guinea pig that I had free ranging and he it was, along with my much loved Ben who lived to a ripe old age of nine, were the rexes that made me fall in love with the breed so much.

There is a very sad story about Ben. He was a chunky tri-coloured boar, belonging to Brenda, a friend of mine who was very deeply into guinea pigs and lived locally. I had known her and her family for about three years when she was suddenly diagnosed as suffering from bone cancer that was terminal. I remember visiting her in hospital a few times and during one of her more lucid periods, when the pain killing drugs were not overwhelming her mind, she asked if I would take on her guinea pigs after she died. Of course I agreed.

"You always did want Ben, didn't you," she pointed out with heavy irony.

"Hm, but I would rather not have got him like this," I told her. She asked if I would take Ben to her funeral and I agreed.

That the old boy went on to live to such a ripe old age, the eldest any guinea pig of mine has ever lived, somehow seemed appropriate. It was as if he was making up for so much of the life that Brenda didn't live for she was only forty one when she died.

For a while I put Ben free range but he didn't seem to settle so he spent the rest of his life with several sows but unfortunately didn't manage to sire any offspring.

By chance, shortly after Ben had begun life with these sows, Teddy arrived. He was a large buff Rex, about eighteen months old and the owners wanted to get rid of him because they said that he had been very nasty to their children, biting one of them. The children in question had come along with their parents and were the most obnoxious, ill mannered little horrors that I had come across in a long time and I remember thinking to myself, "Good for you lad, I hope you bit hard!" There was little doubt in my mind that he had bitten because he had been mishandled.

No doubt as a direct consequence of living with those children, Teddy turned out to be the kind of piggy that didn't suffer fools gladly but he was also not keen on his own kind either. I tried several baby boars with him and even some adult sows but he would have none of it. He even used to rattle his teeth at the sows in their pen when they stood up, hooked their forepaws over the top of the glass and poked their snout at him. He clearly thought that they were on the verge of invading his space!

There was an air of authority about him and he could be very upperty if people tried to pick him up when he was not in a mood for it. For a while I took to calling him the colonel but in the end I settled for just adding the sir name Teddimous.

"Mr Teddimous, stop that!" was a scolding he quite often received when he was rattling his teeth at the girls or at something else that annoyed him such as my slippers, or some other inanimate object! However, though he could be irascible and feisty he was still one of the most laid-back lap piggies I have ever owned. Lap time had to be when he was in the mood for it but when he was he would actually come up and paw at my feet. Once on my lap he would stretch out, front and back legs at full extension and purr like a cat when I stroked him more vibrantly than any other guinea pig I had ever owned.

It was the arrival of Dennis and Dusty, two brother, golden agoutis on the scene that cut short Teddy's free range life with me but carry on with it with a friend of mine who had fallen in love with him. Normally, once a piggy is free range then he is free range for life with me but when I was told that Dusty and Dennis had been free rangers for the whole of their lives, they were two years of age at the time I got them, I jumped at the chance of seeing if I could get a couple of free rangers in my flat.

There was a touch of the beaver in their looks and so much of the 'Hail fellow well met' in their characters. I think that the main reason they didn't fall out when they were set free range in my flat in close proximity with so many sows in the main pen was because of the imbalance of their sex drives. Dennis had one that was at the top of the scale whereas Dusty's would hardly register even at the lower end of it. If there was any 'rumble strutting,' the deep vibrant purring and bottom wriggling that both boars and sows make when they are in the mood for love, I always knew that it would be coming from Dennis. He, it was, who would spend a great deal of his time up on his back legs, forepaws hooked over the glass of the sow pen, chatting up the girls. More often than not, Dusty would be sitting nearby looking at the antics of his brother with an air of distain or bracing himself for the inevitable embrace to come!

Most boars are ambidextrous, so to speak, when it comes to the their choice of the sex their partners and Dusty and Dennis were no exceptions. Having worked himself up and obviously coming to the conclusion that the sows who had hit his 'on' button were unavailable, Dennis would turn away from the pen and rumble his way over to his brother. There would be a couple of sensuous sideswipes, bum to bum, shoulder to shoulder, and he would hop up and happily hump him! Sometimes he got the wrong end and Dusty would tuck his head well down, presumably to avoid nasal or eye penetration!

Not once did I see the slightest gesture of dissent from Dusty, neither was there any signs of enjoyment, Dennis's sexual assault would be met with total indifference or there would be a look of utter resignation. As far as Dusty was concerned this was something that his brother did to him, it didn't last long or cause any permanent damage so what the hell, seemed to be his attitude!

Of all pairs of boars I have owned, I think Dusty and Dennis were the most friendly to one another and were seldom out of one another's company. If one of them came into my living room then it was only a minute or so before the other one would arrive and seek out his brother.

At a very young age they learned the gentle art of sitting upright on their haunches and begging like a pair of dogs for some food. This is not something that many guinea pigs that I have owned have managed to get the hang of. They were certainly the only ones that could hold this stance for any length of time, not that this was very often necessary for my response was usually immediate and the begged for food was supplied.

I had these two lovely boys for about three years. Dennis was the first to go. I found him neatly half mooned in the pen one morning and as in the case of most sudden deaths in guinea pigs that have shown no symptoms of any health problems, a heart attack is probably the way he exited.

Dennis.

Your world was my carpet, bounded by pens of your own kind.
All of them female too, which you could see but not touch.
Cloistered you were, yet free to roam and lust in your mind,
So though you died a virgin it didn't really matter much.

There was always Dusty, available, an obliging brother.
A substitute sow. Who didn't mind the occasional hump or two.
He kept you happy when you wanted him, and sometimes, the

other.

And made him feel useful. A port in a storm, always on cue.

He's in their pen, now you have gone, where you always
                                                    wanted to be.
But happy to see and not touch. Celibate, their perfect guest.
If he's missing you he's not letting on, more stoical than me,
Or perhaps he know you're out to stud at least with Katie and
                                                    the rest.

Watching Dusty wondering about the flat, always looking for his brother, tore my heart out so I put him in the main sow pen where he seemed to be much happier. He remained there, not showing the slightest sexual interest in the sows for about four months. I found him, half mooned in the same way as his brother one morning, quite dead.

Together again.

Have you found him Dusty lad and is he still great fun?
Do you talk of times we had, when you were here with me?
I bet he still creeps up on you and tries to give you one.
I'm sure you let him have his way and sit there patiently.

Tell him that I miss him so, as much as I miss you.
You complimented me each day by making here your home.
I still remember all the warm and funny things you'd do.
The wisest thing I ever did was letting you both roam.

They are there in another clip on the video which featured Doddy and myself doing our stuff, saucy, self assertive and very much at home. It is the way that all of my free rangers have settled so quickly to co-habitation with me, and come to my call, or come to me and scrounge food as their right and due that make them so endearing.

I now come to my current free ranger, Paddington. Like Teddy Tedimous, he is a buff rex. A big bold boy but a very gentle one. He arrived, along with two other boars when they were about five months old. They had belonged to a breeder and as they were not up to show quality they were surplus to requirements, so to speak. As is usually the case with guinea pigs bred by breeders, they were very nervous because being one of hundreds that were kept in small quarters in sheds they had had very little contact with human beings.

I wasn't even going to attempt to keep the three together, so when a friend of mine asked if she could give a home to one of them I readily agreed. I put the remaining two in a pen in my living room where they could get used to the rough and tumble of flat life and hopefully tame down. For the first two weeks they were complete nervous wrecks, scurrying into the furthest corner of their pen whenever I came into the room or made any kind of sudden movement. I think of all the guinea pigs that I have taken in from a breeder, these two were the most nervous and took the longest time to settle down. It was good two months before I could pick them up without the pair of them having an attack of the vapours.

After a couple of months I put them free range and within a couple of days Percy, Paddington's brother, began to get very aggressive towards Paddington. There was no doubt in my mind that it was of a sexual nature, triggered by him having nose to nose access, so to speak, with the sows in the main pen. As someone had already shown a great interest in him and I was determined to keep Paddington free range I rehomed Percy. He is still alive and happy, living with a family who tell me that he has never shown any kind of aggression to any member of the family, confirming my theory that Percy was not a naturally aggressive guinea pig.

I don't think I can call Paddington a solitary boar for in the three years that he has been free ranging he has had about a dozen lady friends. As most of my space has to be reserved for refugees from vets or homeless guinea pigs

113

I seldom breed from my stock or if I do it will be just once to continue a particularly favourite animal's line. In friend Paddington it has simply been a matter of his good looks and lovely temperament, captivating all who meet him.

"Oh dear, he's absolutely adorable, do you think I could bring one of my girls up to see if they would make babies together?" is usually the beginning of yet one more liaison for a happy little lad who is always willing to oblige! To date, only one of these unions has proved fruitless, and we are now up into two figures in the number of ladies who have been in and out of his life!

I am certainly very happy with this arrangement for each time a new lady arrives it means that I shall have a pair of free rangers for up to two months chuntering about the flat. It sometimes takes that long before I am satisfied that the sow in question is up and running well into her term.

It is still necessary for free rangers to have their own open fronted quarters, allowing them to come and go as they please and they are in the kitchen. Initially, when a guinea pig is given the right to free range, it will spend a great deal of time in it's quarters, treating them as a kind of sanctuary from the big wild world of my flat, which must be very intimidating after being confined to an enclosed pen or cage. However, they soon become bolder and begin to explore their surroundings and invariably they will pick out another particular spot in my flat that they will regard as their very own. As soon as they have established their own little bit of personal space I will place down a small mat there for that is where most of their droppings will be deposited. Paddington has made his special spot at the pillow end of my futon. When it is pulled out into the sleeping position it gives him a nice roof about ten inches above his head. I guess he finds it kind of cosy! It also, of course, makes him very close to source all 'all thing bright and edible', myself!

Paddington is one of the all time favourites at G.O.S.H. and when I am seeing new patients, particularly those that may not have had much experience of guinea pigs I always tell them that I have a real live teddy bear in my traveling box. He certainly looks like one and the 'oohs and aah's at the sight of him being hauled out of his compartment are very rewarding. However, as in the school situation there is always one!

Paddington, has picked up a little trick that so many of my other free rangers learned in that he can manipulate me, despite the fact that I am well aware that he is doing it. This trick is so endearing because every time he does it he is confirming the close relationship that always builds up between myself and my free rangers.

Normally, when he wants a titbit, he will come and sit boldly down in front of me and blatantly beg. If this fails he will simply pull at my trouser bottoms. However, there are times when he kind of plays with me. He will cross the room and begin to slow down when he gets level with me, looking about him with an air of great unconcern. Sometimes he will stop completely, and pause to do a bit of grooming, but throughout I will catch him throwing glances in my direction. The aim of the game is to pretend that he is not on the bum but we both know that he is for it always ends up with my getting to my feet with an "OK, Pad, lets see what we can find you" and off I trot into the kitchen. The fact that there is no excitement as the lad trots along behind me to get his just rewards merely shows that he has won again as he knew he would!

I still think it's a bad idea for families to have free rangers for the risks of danger to them is that much higher but for someone living alone and who is willing to put in a bit of time in training both the piggy and themselves, there is nothing quite like having a Fred in your home!

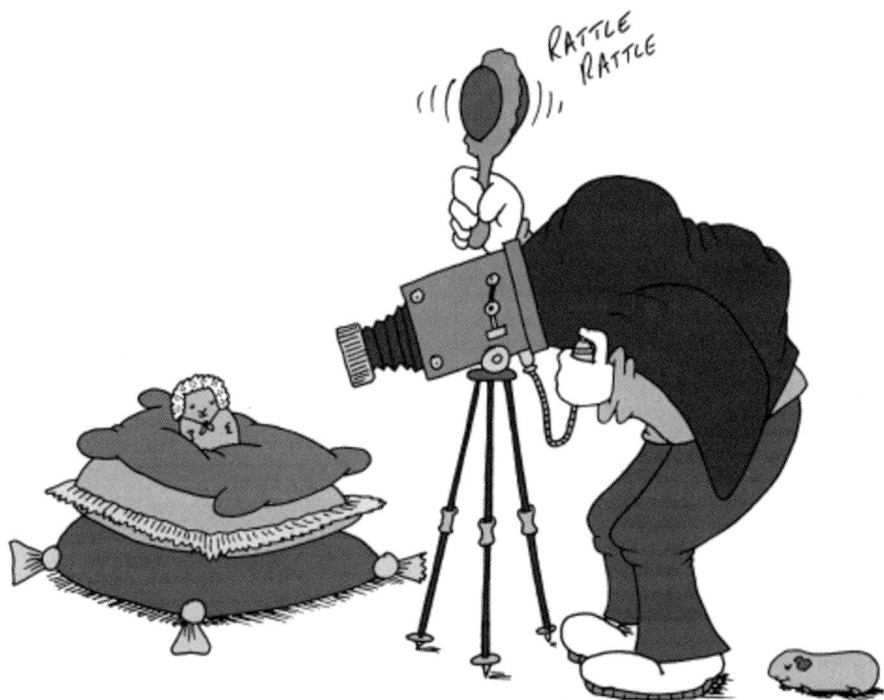

RATTLE RATTLE

Chapter Twelve.

More books to write.

I have a black and white photograph on my wall of Vedra, holding a guinea pig by the name of Willers in her arms. I need it there because the next time I am weeping my heart out when yet one more of my wee friends has died I can be reminded that there is one human being I respect the most in the world who knows just how I feel, for that's how it always hits her when it happens to her.

My daughters, Sarah and Amanda, also understand my tears of course, being great guinea pig fans and owners. At the ages of thirty five and thirty six I am delighted at their refusal to grow up and out of the wee beasties as, sadly so many children seem to.

Willers had a long history of neglect and was brought to the Trust by a lady who decided that if action were not soon taken he would die. She visited the owner, whom she had spoken to many times about the state of Willers and said that as she was going down to the Trust could she take Willers? The owner agreed and Willers came into Vedra's life.

Living in a damp hutch at the bottom of a garden, the fungal skin condition that Willers was suffering from had become systemic and he was in an appalling condition. As the only attention he got was when the owners threw his daily food ration, he was consequently very nervous of human beings.

During the two months that it took to get Willers out of danger and really back onto his feet I witnessed the wonderful phenomenon of him and Vedra bonding. He must have been about three and a half years of age, though he looked much older when he arrived, caked with fungal spores that made a concrete-like overcoat on his skin he was a mess. However, when the hair began to come through, his golden agouti breed began to blossom, not only in looks but in temperament. The owner decided that she did not want the responsibility of looking after him and asked if the Trust would keep him, which suited Vedra and us all very well for we had all become very fond of him.

In my 'What's my guinea pig?' book, I stated that I regarded the agouti breeds as the kind of no nonsense, down to earth breed of the guinea family and Willers was a shining example of this. Despite all that he had suffered in his home and what Vedra had had to put him through, stripping what hair had been left on him and treating the appalling lesions on his skin, he responded by giving her his trust and always rushing to the front of his quarters whenever she passed by. We began to kid Vedra that she and Willers were an item and I know that she felt that it was a compliment to her.

Willers went on to live for another two years, during which time the sight him and Vedra warmed all our hearts. When the end did come I was the first to know.

I had a very early morning telephone call from Vedra. She was in tears and I didn't have to ask what the problem was for we had been aware that Willers was having kidney problems, which were probably due to his age and damage caused during his long illness. Time and illness had simply caught up with the lad.

She asked me if I was coming up to the Trust as arranged the following day and when I told her that I was she asked if I would bury him for her and I readily agreed.

Vedra looked very red eyed and tired when I arrived the following day. We found a quiet spot in a flower bed in the front garden and I soon dug a small grave. When I went in to collect Willers the sight that met my eyes seen had me feeling very weepy. She had just put him in his makeshift coffin, a shoe box. She had wrapped him in one of her best silk scarves, and around his neck was a Saint Christopher's medallion on a thin chain. If that were not enough, when she put the lid on the box written on the top was the message 'Have a nice journey, love Vedra.'

This is a side of Vedra that many people miss and presume is not there. The trouble is that most people who arrive at the Trust are there with their sick animals and what they see is the 'professional' face of this amazing lady, which is focused entirely upon the animal who's health she will be responsible for.

I am very protective towards Vedra as I am to my daughters, even thought they are pretty good at taking care of themselves.

Towards the end of her career as flight attendant. Amanda stuck mainly to short haul work to the continent, which meant that she only had the occasional night away from home, there was no problem about caring for her guinea pigs. Needless to say, as someone who gets vertigo being any higher off the ground than his inside leg measurement, I was very much the worrying 'father.' when she was flying.

On one occasion I wanted to go to her airline and punch the head of the captain of the aircraft she was flying in. By this time, she was a senior air attendant, not a new girl in her first job. I point this fact out to underline the point that the arrogant man with stripes on his sleeve who had learned how to fly a

118

huge modern aircraft was really still a nasty little boy who probably enjoyed tearing the wings off butterflies when he was in short trousers!

One of Amanda's favourite guinea pigs had died and she had, naturally enough being crying for the loss of her small friend. While the rest of the flight crew were kind and understanding about her bleary eyes and sadness, the captain dismissed her concerns with a brusque "Oh don't be silly. It was only a bloody guinea pig."

I am used to this level of lack of compassion for the feelings of others for I now not only come across it in the general public but know that in the main, it is the attitude of far too many veterinary surgeons. That the size of an animal should determine the value put upon it or the feelings of those who love it, says much about the people who think this weird way. To me it reflects a mind that, to quote Oscar Wild, 'know the price of all things but the value of nothing.'

Gathering friends is one of the delightful bonuses of curing guinea pigs, and the misanthropic man that had looked upon his own species with such a jaundiced eye for so many years is much changed. Knowing that the happiness of these friends is much dependent upon the health and welfare of the animals we mutually love is a great spur to my researches and writing. I always keep in mind that they are not as fortunate as me in being able to cope with many ailments that guinea pig flesh is heir to. They have to rely on members of the R.C.V.S., which is not a very good option for either the health of their animals or their bank balances. My books can help them circumvent these people.

One most serious area of ignorance amongst veterinary surgeons is that of the vital business of the reproduction of the species of guinea pigs. The feed-back we used to get led us on many an occasion to question the owner again and establish that he or she really had heard correctly when yet another vet had come out with a piece of nonsense that was either anatomically ridiculous or was like something that came out of the minds of small children when they first questioned where babies came from! Therefore my next book just had to be, 'The sex life of the guinea pig.'

The trigger that made me decide to write it was the arrival of a guinea pig that had a simple breach birth. The owner had luckily been at home when the animal went into labour, had read one of my books, which briefly described the birth process and quickly realized that there was a problem. She had also had had some contact with other owners connected with the Trust and been warned about the reluctance of the vast majority of vets to manually manipulate young from small animals. They much preferred to go straight to the more dangerous and in most cases unnecessary caesarian sections. Also, though the induction drug, Oxytocin is perfectly safe and effective to use in cases of pregnancy inertia, very few vets will use it on guinea pigs, preferring the C section option

Such was the case with the breach birth and the owner had tried three vets, all of whom wished to carry out a C section on the guinea pig. Placing the sow on a towel on my kitchen table, reaching for my trusty tube of KY gel, and squirting and generous amount into the birth canal, within about five minutes I had managed to turn the baby that was breached. It was dead, they usually are if they have been in breach for very long, but the two waiting to come into this breathing world behind it were alive and kicking and popped out in quick succession.

I had by this time manually aided many mothers with this and various other birth problems, my expertise improving with each case. Only on one occasion had I decided that the only option was a C section and luckily the vet I sent it to had the sense to operate right away before the animal became too weak from it's fruitless contractions to with withstand the ordeal. Both mother and babies survived and I was delighted to know that my faith in this particular vet had been rewarded yet once again.

One thing that did please me when I set out upon writing the book was the fact that it would give me a chance to photograph what I regard as the most enchanting time in the life cycle of a guinea pig, littering down! Of course, having learned right from the start through my experience with Squeak, and by this time so many other mother guinea pigs, that there was no way that a sow would perform at my convenience, I had to have a set-up in my living room which, in essence I could then allow me a twenty four hour watching brief, the cameras permanently at the ready.

I partitioned off four feet of the right hand end of the sow pen and divided it into two maternity pens. It took about eight months and a succession of seven pregnant sows before I got all the necessary 'action' shots for sufficient number of slides to illustrate the book.

I have very painful memories every time I look at the most graphic shots that were chosen by my publisher for the book. These were the ones of Evie doing her stuff. She had decided to litter down at about two fifteen one morning. Of course it just had to happen that the previous day I had managed to get a couple of wonderful CD's of live Count Basie performances so that night I had sat there jigging about with more than glass of whiskey or three! I guess I should be thankful that I had not had sufficient alcohol to put me into a deep sleep so when the all too familiar grunt of a Evie having her first contractions managed to get through to my booze befuddled brain, I did manage to wake up. Dehydration was beginning to set in, I had a mouth like the bottom of a parrot's cage and a head, which a hundred aspirins couldn't put right!.

Evie had already got one of her babies out by the time I positioned myself with the camera and begun shooting. Luckily, mother guinea pigs are not at all disturbed by flashing or noisy camera mechanisms. To take a different angled shot of baby number three emerging, I leaned forward and twisted my body. The all too familiar click in the lower lumber region of my back, followed by an equally familiar shooting pain, heralded two weeks of walking about with the posture of a ruptured duck and wincing in pain at the slightest bend in my back. For the many like-sufferers of that well known phenomenon of 'Putting the back out' I do not have to explain any further what kind of agony I was in!

If someone else had been in that room during the following twenty minutes, and they had had a camera upon me as I crawled about on hands and knees trying to continue my photographic mission they would have managed to get some very precious shots indeed! I do remember at one stage, despite my pain, collapsing in a heap in a fit of the giggles, interspersed with gasps of agony when I had happened to catch sight of my self in a nearby full length mirror. There I was in all my naked glory, ashen, bleary eyed, what little hair still on my head, tousled, on my hands and knees and clutching a state of the art Pentax camera. I muttered something like, 'Gurney what you go through for your art!'

Here and there, in the main pen, I caught sight of one of the sows, lying there, eyeing me, in puzzlement. A rustle from just above my head drew my attention the boar pens above. Alex was leaning over the glass-front, one eye visible through the unruly mob of his Peruvian fringe, looking at me speculatively.

"You can keep your big nose out of it for a start," I admonished, grumpily.

He began pawing at the top of the glass excitedly, obviously misinterpreting my moaning for some kind of offer of some kind of juicy tit-bit. I ignored him and got back to the business in hand.

It must have been about an hour later that I got to bed because I not only needed shots of the actual birth, I wanted ones of the cleaning, nursing and the shot that I knew had to come. These would be of the great moment when mother and all snuggle down together to rest after the ordeal of making their entrance into this living breathing world. On more than one occasion, I am not ashamed to say that this wonderful sight has brought tears to my eyes, and always the ironic remark, 'That's it my little ones, there you are, behaving like animals!'

If I remember rightly we used slides from three of the other births that took place during the time my maternity pens were in use. One other of these births were in the early hours, the rest during the day.

Normally, I do not isolate my sows from the main pack when they are due to litter down. I did, once upon a time for I had been told that this was the way it was done and that the mother and babies could be harmed by other pack members. If I had sat and thought about this for a minute or so I would have released what a ridiculous notion this was. Why would other pack members harm those of it's own species that were engaged in the vital business of the reproduction of the species! It was only after I had seen some of the appallingly cramped condition of some irresponsible breeders who had experienced this phenomenon that I realized how this myth had come about. Any over crowded animals can resort to this kind of behaviour!

The other deciding factor was experiencing a couple of cases where my sows had littered down in the main pen earlier than I had expected so I had not had chance to segregate them. In the first case there had been a couple of other sows lying close to her and neither took the slightest interest what so ever other than the very briefest of sniffs in the direction of the action until after she had delivered her litter, thoroughly cleaned all her young and snuggled them under her. Then, one after another, they slowly got to their feet, crossed slowly to the mother and babes, gave them a quick look over and a more thorough sniffing and then resumed their places. There was no sign of alarm in either the mother or the babies.

In the other case, though it didn't happen in the main pen but a small one with three sows and a boar in it, the sows having been brought to me specifically for breeding with my boar, I had the chance to watch the behaviour of a boar when one of his sows littered down and what a delightful sight it turned out to be. I can't be sure that all boars behave this way with their littering sows for this was the only time I witnessed such a phenomenon for I normally take out my boars at least a week before littering down. This is because the sow comes into season shortly after birth and a boar would try and mate with her again.

Once more the other sows in the pen took very little interest in what was going on but as soon as the first baby was out, the boar immediately went over and assisted the mother in cleaning it and continued doing so with the rest of the litter. Once the cleaning was completed and the sow and young had settled down he moved away, the other sows behaved in the same way as those I had seen in the main pen with the littering mother. I felt quite bad about removing the boar but I knew that within an hour or so the sow would come into season.

I have one sow, Treacle who was also featured in the book littering down, who now behaves like the main sow pen midwife! In this case, though she is the only one I had ever owned that has behaved in this manner, I have heard that this kind of behaviour has been witnessed by other people with experience of sows living in packs so it is not unique to my own sow. As soon as she hears that familiar grunt of a sow experiencing her first contraction, she will be at her side P.D.Q. She will assist in the cleaning and nursing of the young but it is very noticeable that she will always push the babies back to the mother after she is satisfied that the business has been completed. She will usually stay close to the mother for about forty eight hours and continue nursing the young. There is an air of authority about her, which doesn't seem to be resented by the mother who seems to welcome the attention. I am sure that this is because Treacle seems to make it clear by all her actions that she makes no claim to the babies as her own. At the end of this time Treacle will leave the mother and babies alone and go back to business as usual with the rest of the pack.

Little did I know that 'The sex life of the guinea pig,' was going to take me to Washington DC in the States, a couple of years after I had submitted the text to my publisher. This book signing visit was to cement a growing relationship with the many wonderful American friends I had been making via my books.

It was about this time that I took up the new toy the WWW. I stayed with it for about a year then gave it up. Leaving aside the hour and a half each day it took to answer all the e mails I received regarding the husbandry and veterinary care of guinea pigs, I was mighty disappointed discovering the same slavish forelock tugging to those with letters after their names a great disappointment. It short, the WWW did the very opposite from what it claimed to do, provide a venue for the exchange of new ideas and information. Those on the various guinea pig websites seemed more interested in the fact that I was letterless than in any kind of new ideas I or anyone else outside the establishment veterinary circles may have come up with, particularly if they went against the holy grail of accepted veterinary practice. The pettiness and back biting that went on finally made me sign off and I am very unlikely to sign on again.

There is a website still running on my behalf which has two sections in it, Vetcare and Vetwatch. The first to is give information for those who have open minds, the second is to alert the public to the real state of the kind of service the British public has to put up with from the R.C.V.S,s monopoly.

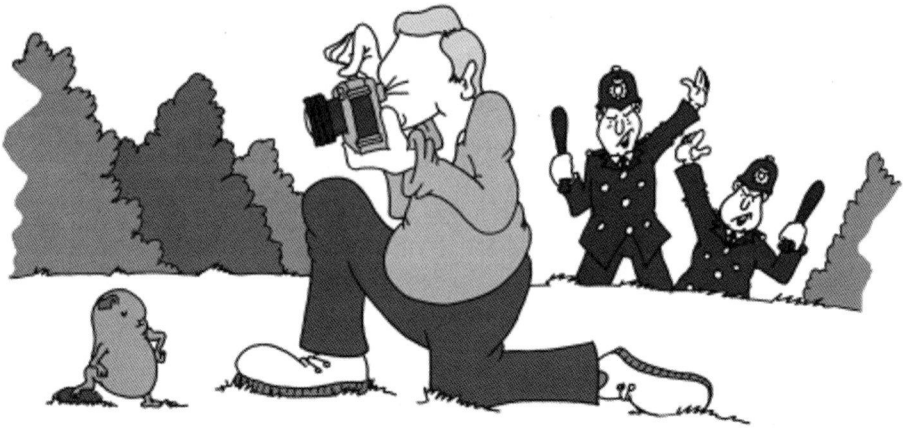

Chapter Thirteen.

Oh the children, and the piggies the park.

I wrote in one of my books that guinea pigs are a handful for adults and an armful for children. I think I was trying to make the point that they are both child and adult sized! I also wrote that for a man of my age to be able to experience the same feeling, for the same reason, at the same time as a child was just has to be something special. However, guinea pigs have the ability to bring out the child in adults and this Chapter is about the 'children' in the park as well as the children in the hospital.

It is the ability of children to say it as it is, which makes them such a wonderful source of anecdotes. I think the most up front child I ever met was Saun. She may have had a Welsh name but from the way she spoke she was a bright little cockney sparrow. She was about eight or nine years of age and had spent much of her life in the hospital. The only thing I did know about her was that she was unable to eat normally and had to be fed intravenously. It was only after I had been visiting her for quite a while that I was told that she was liable to die young. Whether she knew this I do not know but if she did she did not brood and was one of the most chatty, happy children I have ever met.

Another volunteer told me that one day when she was visiting Saun the lunch trolley arrived and without thinking she asked her what she was having for lunch. The volunteer told me that before she had actually finished the sentence she realized what a big gaff she had made and felt absolutely terrible. She needn't have worried for Saun brushed the remark aside with a bright and breezy, "Don't be daft, I don't eat, do I!"

Saun adored all my guineas and we usually ended up with three or four in the bed with her. I arrived one morning when her nurse was just removing one of the drips tubes and was setting up some other monitoring device and attaching the wires from it to Saun.

"Hold on a minute, till the nurse has finished with you," I said, alarmed at the way Saun was getting excited and bouncing about on the bed, tubes and wires attached, in eager anticipation of some quality guinea pig time.

The nurse eventually sorted her out and pulled the sheet over her, which Saun immediately kicked off.

"Saun, you've got no knickers on," scolded the nurse.

Saun, turned to the nurse, put out her tongue then calmly stated the facts of the case "It's only Peter, he's seen my bum before, haven't you?" and Indeed I had.

On more than one occasion I had arrived when the nurse was engaged in some procedure which meant clothes or equipment were being changed. Usually I back out and wait till things like this are completed, respecting the patient's right to privacy but Saun always managed to see us and had no time for such adult sensibilities.

My favourite wards are those that deal with the heart transplants and general heart surgery. The term bravery is used to describe the way the children cope but honestly do not think that the children think of what they have to go through is any big deal. With one or two very rare exceptions the children have an attitude of business as usual.

I particularly remember one little girl who had had a heart transplant who

I am sure was deliberately winding me up. The first time I saw her was not long after the transplant so she was lying there with load of monitoring and support gear attached to her but as 'with it' as a healthy child when she saw the wee ones.

"Doggy," says she.

"Guinea pig," says I.

Each Tuesday for the next four weeks, by which time she was ready to be transferred to her local hospital, it was the same thing. She is insisted that my wee beasties were doggies while I maintained they were guinea pigs.

By this time, of course, she was detached from all the medical paraphernalia and at the time when she delivered what was to be her parting shot she was sitting in her father's arms.

As I put the guineas back in their traveling box just before leaving I paused with Paddington in my arms, held him up and looked her right in the eyes.

"Guinea pig," I said, very firmly.

The mere trace of a smile crossed her face, she inclined her head and gave me a very old fashioned kind of look.

"Guinea ....doggy," she said, with a slight interrogative lift to her voice.

I swear she knew all the time and had simply been winding me up.

I held Paddington higher and looked at him as though I was examining him anew.

"Hm! On second thought perhaps he is a guinea doggy," I told her.

I said to her father that old fool that I could be I was not as silly as to have not have learned the lesson that when a women compromises with your you after a long dispute you damn well compromise too, if you have any sense in your head!

Most of the children, or leastwise those that I see, seem to recover and get back onto their feet very quickly after heart surgery. The first time they will be flat on their backs with all the monitors and life support equipment plugged into them. It is not at all unusual, that when I visit them a week later they are sitting up free of the bulk of the equipment and are bright as buttons.

One little girl I saw, about two and a half weeks after her transplant was bouncing up and down on her bed when I arrived. Her parents had specially asked for me to visit as she had piggies of her own. We quickly settled some piggies on a towel on the bed and she petted and fed them, chattering to them all the time. Suddenly she looked up at me and said, "I've got a new heart."

"Is it a good one?" I asked, trying to be as blasé about it as she was.

"I bloody sight better than the old one," she replied, with a grin, and turned her attention to the wee ones again.

I always take up nursing mother guinea pigs and their young, and on these occasions allow much more time for I know that I shall be there for much longer. The nurses tend to steal the babies, putting them in their uniform pockets and doing their own piggy visiting to their particular favourite patients. However, on one occasion one of the doctors got in on the act. I had been visiting a little boy who was a long term patient and when a beautiful cream sow by the name of Nedine gave birth to two of Paddington's babies I took her and her brood to see the little boy.

I put Nedine and her babes into the boy's cot and his mother and I settled down to watch. Not unusually, as soon as mum and babes were settled in the warm woolen coverlet they did what came naturally and begun to suckle. The little boy watched, fascinated and about a minute later one of his doctors arrived. If the boy was fascinated then the doctor was transfixed. The mother and myself were completely forgotten the boy and the doctor watched Nedine doing her stuff.

"I think we could go and get ourselves a cup of tea," I remarked, loudly.

"Hm, good idea," said the doctor, half turning. "Leave us boys to play!"

I did, of course get to know the adorable little Bosnian girl, Irma who was an inspiration. She was a big fan of Katie, one of my beautiful Peruvian sows and had pictures of her round her bed. I told her that if she got pregnant and had babies I would definitely name one after her.

Each time I saw that child, paralyzed from the neck down because of the crass stupidity of adults and was warmed by her ever welcoming wide eyed smile I used to think to myself, "Kid, you have more guts than all those armies put together!"

The enduring memory I have of her is of her driving her specially constructed electric propelled chair, which she operated with all the skill of a grand prix driver via a small joy stick rigged under her chin, at the last Christmas party she attended in the staff canteen before she died.

The "children" in the park, St James' park to be precise, were a different kettle of fish but delighted me the same.

Apart from the way the park is laid out and the number of wonderful, large trees dotted about, which had wonderfully gnarled trunks and over ground roots which made ideal backgrounds for piggy pics, it was the variety of nationalities I met there that made it just that more enjoyable.

These people soon put me right on the various names they had for guinea pigs in their own language. Though some of these people had no idea what kind of animals I was cradling in my lap, I usually took two, quite a few of them had either owned guinea pigs when they were young or still had them. Needless to say, the Americans were the most likely to be current guinea pig owners and I was not at all surprised for I got the most feed back from the States from my books and knew that they were into them in a big way.

As for the piggies themselves, they were not at all worried by the big wide open spaces of the park and the vast amount of people who petted them. Obviously, I only took guineas that were naturally laid back and the two most popular by far were my adorable cream boars, Simon and Garfunkel, with Dandy coming up a close second. It was while I was photographing Dandy that I am sure that I threw huge scare into the police responsible for protecting number ten Downing street.

Normally, any photography that I needed to do in the park was done either in the afternoon or more often, in the evening when the sun was low in the sky and more mellow and setting behind Buckingham Palace. However, my

130

favourite building was the old Clive building, now the National Statistic Office, which is on the west side of the park. I had this bee in my bonnet about getting a shot of Dandy sitting on the high curbing round the lawns that surround this building but having the sun rising behind him.

To set the scene, I think I had better point out that about three days before I decided to get up early and down to the site just before dawn the IRA had thrown a bomb over the wall into the back garden of Number 10 Downing Street!

I duly arrived and after trying several positions decided that the best way to get my shots was from the left of the Clive building. That way could get more of the building in by composing the picture so that Dandy was in the left hand side of the frame and the bulk of the building in the right.

The promise of a cloudless day and warm summer weather was realized as the sun begun to rise and shine through the trees and the gaps between the buildings in the middle distance directly behind where I was to pose Dandy, one of which was----------number ten Downing street!

As soon as I had made sure that there were some bits of greenery on the curbing for Dandy to nibble on, posing him was no trouble at all. It was about thirty seconds after I had sprawled out on the pavement and begun to site the camera and adjust the settings that things begun to happen, and happen quickly and very noisily indeed.

There was a screech of tyres in the roadway behind, and to the left of me, which froze me for a brief second. I eventually turned, in time to see two very large police officers in very bulky jackets getting out of a high performance police vehicle and baring down on me and Dandy. He, by the way, was not at all phased and got on with the number one priority of feeding his face!

These police officers were John Wayne sized and with the same kind of determined look on their faces, arms hanging loosely by their sides, ready no doubt to reach in for what ever heavy artillery they were carrying that made the jackets so bulky! It didn't take me more than a second or so to realize what this was about. I had a particular fondness for all the mainly government buildings

131

at that side of the park and appreciated the way that though all had surveillance cameras on them covering the whole of the area they were not obtrusive.

Obviously what the camera's had seen was a man laying flat on the ground, directly in line with Number ten and aiming something in the mellow glow of the dawning sun!

I got to my feet, now acutely embarrassed, and floundering for something to say to explain myself and came out with a very lame, "Oh, all the park police all know me, I'm here all the time," and indeed they did. There was a very pregnant pause and a bit of a hard stare from one of the officers.

"Ah, but you are not park police, are you!" I said in an even more lame voice.

"No Sir, we are not" the officer replied, succinctly.

By this time they had drawn level with me and caught site of Dandy.

"That's a guinea pig, isn't it" said the officer who had put me right about the kind of policeman he was!

"Hm, I wanted to get a shot of him with the Clive building in the background at sunrise," and hastily begun to gather up my paraphernalia.

The police officer looked at his colleague, there was a brief shrug of his shoulders, then he gestured me to carry on.

"No law against it as far as I know," he said, turning back to the car. As they drove away I could see that the pair of them were laughing. I have often speculated whether this was just relief that I wasn't what I appeared to be or at the thought of everyone pressing the panic button on account of a wee beastie having his picture taken!

Chapter fourteen.

The American Way.

As I was finishing the Sex life book I had an offer from the English publisher, Harper Collins that I could not resist. They were bringing out a new series of pet care books and asked if I would be interested in being commissioned to write the one about guinea pig care. I jumped at it for by this time there had been so much more that Vedra and I had learned about our subjects.

By this time Vedra had moved to Alconbury and the C.C.T. had become a guinea pig hospital specializing in research into all rodent medicine. Needless to say with access to the kind of expertise that she now had, and what I had been learning about alternative medicine, I was able to put the most up to date information about the proper veterinary care of guinea pigs.

Up until the Collins book I had provide all the photographs for my books and I have to admit that I was a little put out the news that though they wanted to use a few of mine, in the main they would employ a profession wild life photographer. However, when I saw the way he worked and the early proofs of his skills, I bowed to a superior photographer and I was delighted with the results when the book was published.

By this time I had the grand total of four vets in London whom I could refer owners to, confident that they would not be ripped off financially and who's small animal skills had been proved on many occasions to my satisfaction or to the opinions of people who had used their services. However, if anything, in the main, the cases of veterinary gross incompetence, unnecessary and life threatening surgery and outrageous over charging went on a pace. Little did I know that I was soon to see how they did things in another country!

I had been to quite a few books signing venues and thoroughly enjoyed them for it gave me a chance to put faces to many people who wrote or phoned me and to meet new readers of my books. Early in 2000 I did a book singing on the John Ogbourne's Winking Cavy store stand at the Doncaster show and it was then that he first muted the idea of a trip out to the States for a book signing in the USA. While I was not too happy about the thought of the air trip, not only would it be good for the promotion of my books, which were very popular in the States, I really wanted to meet some of the Americans with whom I had been corresponding.

At the Doncaster show with me, signing copies of her own work, was Caroline, a brilliant illustrator who, like so many of the friends I have made, came to me in desperation after a white coat had got it wrong with one of her beloved guinea pigs. We had become good friends over a couple of years and to my delight she was invited on the Washington, making the trip far more pleasant.

As things turned out, the Sex life book came out a couple of months after the Harper Collins one, even though it had been written almost eighteen months earlier. Right up to a day before we left from Heathrow the pressure was on when I spent two days with a camera crew filming a piece of a new T.V. series, and a morning when I was the guest, along with Paddington and one of the many loves in his life on the T.V. programme Big Breakfast.

The new series was basically about people who had adapted their homes in unique ways, or lived unusual kind of lives. Of all the things I have done for T.V. this was the hardest work to do but most rewarding in that it told it as it was, showing what twenty four hours of my life with the wee ones was really like.

Jason Byrne, a stand up comedian, was the front man and the producer proved right in his remarks when he first came to have a look at the flat and have a chat about the series, when he said, 'You and Jason will be great together.' We hit it off right away and got along very well, spending a great deal of the time laughing our socks off. Though we spent almost a day over on Clapham common filming, it was edited out of the final programme. However, I gave the TV crew a good laugh when I related to tale of Chipper's ghost during the filming.

The particular part of the Common where my supply of summer grass comes from is a kind of wood copse on the east side also happens to be quite a notorious Gay cruising area, one where a particular government minister came to grief there a few years after the event occurred that I am about to relate! The attraction for me is the grass which, unlike on the rest of the common, is seldom cut and remains fresh and green because of scrub and tree cover the copse gets throughout any hot spells, thus keeps the ground moist.

When Chipper was alive I used to take him with me and put him down to do a bit of 'pick it yourself' while I cut the grass for the rest of the mob for the following day's breakfast, chatting to him as I worked. After he died I kind of carried on chatting to his ghost. I have since discovered that many guinea pig fixated people carry on conversations with their long dead pets so flaky I maybe but I am in good company!

One morning, as I was crouched, cutting away in the copse there was an interrogative "Yes?" from just in front and slightly above me. I looked up to see a man about my own age wearing only a very tight, very short, pair of denim shorts standing by a small bush.

Embarrassed at having been caught at what must have looked and sounded like me talking to myself I hastily explained, "Oh sorry, I was talking to my guinea pig." As soon as the words left my mouth I knew that they had been replaced by my foot!

The chap peered at the ground about me and I immediately dug a bigger hole for me to step into with, "Oh, no. He's dead. He died years ago I just ...." I didn't bother finishing the sentence, it seemed rather pointless for it wasn't situation that I could ever retrieve!

The look on the poor chap's face said it all, as he quickly moved back behind the bush. "And they call me queer!"

The Big Breakfast, which we had been on many years before, apart from being very good promotion for the Sex life book, was another opportunity to up the profile of the piggies. I have always got a kick from this aspect my work. It is much the same in the States and I entirely agree with a comment an American made, 'It's about time someone said it for the little guys in the pet world!"

I landed in the U.S.A. with the clothes that I stood up in and three pounds sterling in my pocket! Luckily I had given Caroline my flight tickets and my passport. I only had hand luggage and when I put it through the x ray machine at Heathrow I thought it went straight onto the aircraft but apparently I was supposed to pick it up as it came out of the other end! After three days of e mailing and phoning, I gave up trying to get British Airways to forward the luggage, which had been found and placed in the lost property office. Luckily, Caroline had her international credit card and she bankrolled me during the trip.

John Ogbourne who was the main motive force in organizing the trip and flew over with us had made arrangements to hire a car and drove Caroline and myself out to Springfield some fifteen miles out of Washington to the family we were staying with during our trip.

Judi, the lady of the house greeted us by saying, "There is only one rule while you are staying in this house and that is that you never ask for anything you just help yourself." This was our first taste of American hospitality and it is the kind of warmth we received from everyone we met during our stay.

The house was split level in a lovely, leafy neighborhood but the real bonus for us was walking through the front door and seeing and meeting all the wonderful animals. There were three rabbits that were free rangers. Two bucks and a doe. The doe, who was referred to as the tart, used to commute between the bucks who lived in different rooms. All were neutered so there was no danger of a rabbit population explosion and the ménage a trio seemed to work out very well, the bucks sticking strictly to their own rooms.

Judi ran a registered guinea pig refuge and I was delighted to discover that the room I was to sleep in had wall to wall pens full of guinea pigs so I would be very much at home. However, the predominant creature in this household was Oscar, a magnificent African gray Parrot who had his huge cage, it was more the size of a garden gazebo than a cage, situated in the spacious living room. In essence, he only spent the nights in, being released each morning and climbing on top where he spent the day. However, he never did manage to do what Judi hoped he would, and I quote her. "I just hope he picks up Caroline's lovely laugh and the way you Brits say gorgeous!"

A guinea pig extravaganza was held at a large hall and I think it was one of the most enjoyable days of my life for the place was full of piggy people and their wee ones. I got writers cramp signing copies of my books and a sore throat exchanging guinea pig stories. As for the piggy guests, they were of course absolutely superb. On the morning of the extravaganza I fell in the shower and spent the whole day with my right knee twice as large as normal, grimacing whenever I put too much weight on it and limping about like Long John Silver. However, nothing could spoil that very memorable day and the lovely people I met who all treated me as though I was just a long lost friend of many years standing.

Like it is in England, I quickly learned that the range of people hooked on the addictive wee beasties was very varied. The one great things that they all had in common was an ability to talk and enthuse about their animals and be as proud of them as I was of mine. However, the big lesson from the States was taught me when I spent a morning with Judi's vet.

Judi had told me that her vet, Valerie, would probably invite us in to watch her doing the two spaying and two neutering surgical jobs that had to be performed on the four guinea pigs that she was taking there. For a start, the idea that a British vet would invite a client to watch him or her work was of course one that would not even be entertained! Not for any clinical reason but to maintain the 'big mystery' of professionals at work, and of course the fear that they may foul up in front of their clients!

I had seen both these surgical procedures performed before but the way Valerie worked was a sheer joy. She was quick, efficient and had no time for drama about it all. The other main difference between this American vet and her British counterpart was her attitude towards her staff and in particular towards her veterinary nurses, to whom it was clear that she delegated far more responsibility than any British vet would when it came to clinical procedures. There was none of this old stuffy British, 'God' vet and mere veterinary nurse, they worked as a team and the mutual respect they had for one another's skills was clearly evident.

The proof of the pudding was in her record with Judi alone. In the previous year Valerie had performed over a hundred and thirty of these operations and not a single guinea pig had suffered any ill effects from either the surgery or the anaesthesia. I would dearly love to hear of an English vet, other than those working for the Trust or the four in the whole of London that I have any faith in, with anywhere near that kind of record.

After Valerie had finished working on the guinea pigs she invited us to watch her work on a couple of dogs a rabbit and a cat.

Around twelve we were calmly asked, "Hey, have you guys eaten yet? 'cause we are about to send out for some pizzas" and we both accepted her invitation to join her and some of her staff for a lunch break. Once again Judi assured me that this wasn't just because I was there, but her vet kind of made a habit of this. The notion that this open friendliness could happen in an English veterinary surgery is, of course out of the question!

By the time I retuned home I had not only again put many faces to the names of e mails but made very many more friends. Little did I know that these friends were to put their money where their 'friendship was', so to speak a few months later.

Early in the new year the hot water cylinder gave up the ghost. According to my tenancy agreement the repair of this system was supposed to be a number one priority, which had to be put right within twenty-four hours. It took three months, the employment of a solicitor, a press campaign in the local paper, and letters from people all over the world to the leader of Lambeth council before it finally gave in and made the repair. The reason for the delay? The roughy, toughie plumbers working for the contractors who were responsible for these repairs said they would not work with the odour of the guinea pigs.

As anyone who keeps these animals knows, guinea pigs are practically odourless. The local press arranged for a private plumber to come in and give his opinion and an estimate of the cost of repair. In the article in the next edition he stated that the place was clean, and there was no odour at all and he could see no reason why the work could not be carried out.

My American friends found out about what was going on via the Winking cavy store and raised, along with supporters in this country and all over the world, over £500 to help pay my legal costs which left about two hundred and fifty pound which they all agreed I could donate to GOSH. Needless to say I am still awaiting compensation from the council for it's gross breach of duty of repair, a year later!

Chapter fifteen

Role reversal.

The rest of the year was reasonably uneventful, apart from the great honor of not only having a new Olga De Olga book dedicated to me, but actually being a character in it called Mr Gee. My Harper Collins book was translated into French. Most pleasing of all was the number of vets who began seeking our advice, and I found myself teaching several of them our none anaesthetic dental techniques. I up dated 'Piggy potions' for a second print run, and 'What's my guinea pig' went into a second run. However, in the early in 2001 I began to get health problems and by the summer time they were symptomatic of a bowel problem developing which, needless to say, as my sister had died of cancer of the bowel, and this kind of thing can be genetic, myself and my doctor became ever so slightly concerned about. There followed so many tests with all manner of investigative tubes shoved in all manner of orifices! A mass was finally found in my descending colon in September and an appointment was made for abdominal surgery at St Thomas', where I had had my cancerous kidney removed some eleven years earlier.

The surgery took place on the 14th December and I had to stay in hospital over Christmas. Lucky, Sue, who now runs a new website, moved into my flat and took over the care of the wee ones so a great concern was taken care of. Needless to say the support and encouragement I received from the guinea pig fraternity all over the world was a wonderful. It confirmed what I had learned very early on in my life with these adorable animals, which was that piggy people are nice people, as was another long held opinion. It was that whatever they pay nurses it is not enough for their unceasing care and dedication.

Shortly after my surgery, and close to Christmas, a new nurse on the ward came over to my bed and asked if I was the Peter Gurney who wrote the guinea pig books. When I replied in the affirmative she asked if she could bring Hannah, her daughter to see me as she was a big guinea pig fan. That night Hannah, her pig tails with some tinsel in them as she had been in the school play, arrived with photos of her piggies and her mother left us to have some serious guinea pig talk. As Hannah and her mother left the ward, some time later, I reflected that I may not have had real live piggies to hold, as the children had during the eleven years that I had been visiting them, chatting to a child who valued them as much as I did was pretty good substitute!

Sadly, a couple of days after I returned, my adorable Paddington died of septicemia but he did leave me a parting gift, a litter of four. Unfortunately only one survived, a sow whom I just had to call Lucky. As soon as I was recovered enough to feel that I could go out and about again my first real trip out was to GOSH with Wilma and her baby, Lucky. I wanted to let them know that after my Chemo therapy that I would resume normal service on the guinea pig visiting front in a couple of months time.

Walking through the main entrance of GOSH after, what for me had felt like an age, was very good medicine. However, it only got better for I found myself subjected to many hugs from many gorgeous nurses. It's tough work but I guess some one has got to do it! I got the distinct impression that we had been missed. Wilma and Lucky also got their fair share of hugs and one little boy quite forget the pain of teething, along with his medical problem to contend with, when I put the pair down on his bed.

I got a special hug from Jill, one of the chaplain's at GOSH and I asked her to thank the 'Man' when she spoke to him that night. She told me that she was sure that she was only one of many who had been praying for me.

I left that place with my feet two feet above the ground but I think I have been a

little that way since the first guinea pig came into my life all those years ago. They have proved to be a catalyst that has made my life bloom and flower into something which I value far more than when it was bereft of the wee beasties.

As I end this book, Jasper and Jake, two of Paddington's many offspring, are sitting lying on the carpet, having settled down to being free rangers far quicker than any other of their predecessors. They are already beginning to sit up and 'beg pretty please' when they think they can get some titbit from myself or any visitors.

I can only end by saying a big thank you to them and all of their kind, which naturally includes the two legged variety, for enhancing my life and adding so much colour and delight into each day that I live of it.

Peter Gurney   18.1.02

Other Books by Peter Gurney

Title	Publisher
The Proper Care of Guinea Pigs	TFH
Piggy Potions	TFH
What's My Guinea Pig	TFH
The Sex Life of Guinea Pigs	TFH
Guinea Pig Family Pet Guide	Collins

Available from good bookshops and

The Winking Cavy Store   www.winking-cavy.co.uk